TOP FITNESS EXPERTS AND ATHLETES PRAISE JOYCE L. VEDRAL

"I recommend all of Joyce's books to my patients because they provide the most effective workout with the least danger of injury. Her latest, BOTTOMS UP!, especially stands out in that it provides alternative exercises for those who suffer from back and knee trouble."

—Jack Barnathan,
Doctor of Chiropractic, Chairman, Nassau County
Council of Physical Fitness

"As a personal trainer, I am happy that my work is made simple for those who suffer from cellulite. I give BOTTOMS UP! to my clients, ask them to read it, and then I put them on the program. In a matter of months, they are thrilled with the results."

—Gus Stephanidis, Mr. Greece

"Whether you're a pro or a beginner, you can use this book to burn maximum fat and at the same time shape muscle."

—Bev Francis,
IFBB World Pro Bodybuilding Champion,
author of *Bev Francis' Power Bodybuilding*

"BOTTOMS UP! is the answer—not only for the young and out of shape, but for those over forty, fifty, and sixty. Joyce Vedral gives a no-nonsense workout that not only replaces atrophied muscle and gives new shape to the body, but strengthens and thickens weakening bone. I recommend the book to every one of my clients."

—Lud Shusterich,
World Powerlifting Record holder and member of
the All Time Greats Bodybuilding Hall of Fame

"Joyce takes my time-tested principle of the superset and applies it from the bottom up—for a workout that will produce dramatic results—by burning maximum fat and reshaping and building muscle in record time."

—Joe Weider,
publisher of *Shape, Muscle and Fitness,*
and *Men's Fitness*

"Joyce is a role model for women half her age and an inspiration to us all."
—Tanya Knight,
Miss International and
"Gold" on *American Gladiators*

"You get the benefit of an aerobic workout while doing a bodybuilding routine."
—Andy Sivert,
Mr. International, Mr. North America

BOTTOMS UP!

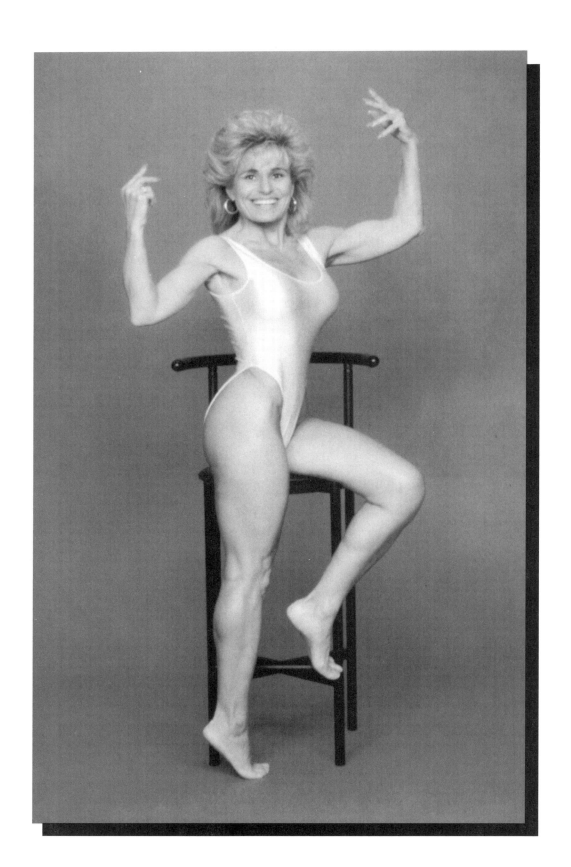

BOTTOMS UP!

The Total-Body Workout from the Bottom Up
From Cellulite to Sexy—in 24 Workout Hours

JOYCE L. VEDRAL, Ph.D.

WARNER BOOKS

A Time Warner Company

A NOTE FROM THE PUBLISHER

The ideas, procedures, and suggestions contained in this book are not intended as a substitute for consulting with your physician. All matters regarding your health require medical supervision.

Copyright © 1993 by Joyce L. Vedral, Ph.D.
All rights reserved.

Warner Books, Inc., 1271 Avenue of the Americas, New York, NY 10020

A Time Warner Company

Printed in the United States of America
First Printing: July 1993
10 9 8 7 6 5

Library of Congress Cataloging-in-Publication Data

Vedral, Joyce L.
    Bottoms up! / Joyce L. Vedral.
       p.   cm.
    Includes bibliographical references.
    ISBN 0-446-39421-1
    1. Reducing exercises.   2. Physical fitness for women.   I. Title.
RA781.6.V429   1993
646.7'5'082—dc20   92-28685
                                         CIP

Book design by Giorgetta Bell McRee
Cover design by Diane Luger
Cover photo by Don Banks
Black and white photos by Don Banks
Hair and makeup by Jodi Pollutro
Cover bathing suit by Nicole's Perfect Fit
Workout leotards by Denise Ko-fe of Ko-fe of California
Gym shoes by Reebok International

To all of us—the women who are bound and determined to have the best body possible, from the bottom up, so that we can free the highest part of our beings, the mind, and concentrate on achieving goals and living our lives to the fullest!

ACKNOWLEDGMENTS

To Joann Davis, for your endless enthusiasm and astute editing.

To Jeanmarie LeMense, for your constant and efficient attention to the details.

To Diane Luger and Jackie Merri Meyer for your expert treatment of the cover and artwork.

To Larry Kirshbaum, Nanscy Neiman, and Ellen Herrick, for your continual enthusiasm and support.

To Joe and Betty Weider, for inventing and promoting the training principles used in this book and by the champions, and for your wonderful magazines: *Muscle and Fitness, Shape, Men's Fitness,* and *Flex.*

To Don Banks for your superior photography.

To Jodi Pollutro of Mike & Me in Manhattan for your wonderful artistry in hair and makeup.

To Carol Acker, for helping me in a hundred ways.

To Nicole Gangi of Nicole's Perfect Fit of Glen Cove, Long Island, New York, for designing the cover and inside bathing suits, and for giving me the perfect fit.

To Ken's Fitness Centre in Farmingdale, Long Island, for providing a peaceful, powerful place to work out.

To Denise, designer of Ko-fe of Los Angeles, California, for creating the perfect leotard for the exercise photographs.

To Joan Mikus, administrator, and Dr. David Lehr and Dr. David Bauer, co-directors of the Pritiken Longevity Center in Miami Beach, for the wonderful life-giving fitness program offered at their facility.

To family and friends for your continual love and support.

CONTENTS

BOTTOMS UP!

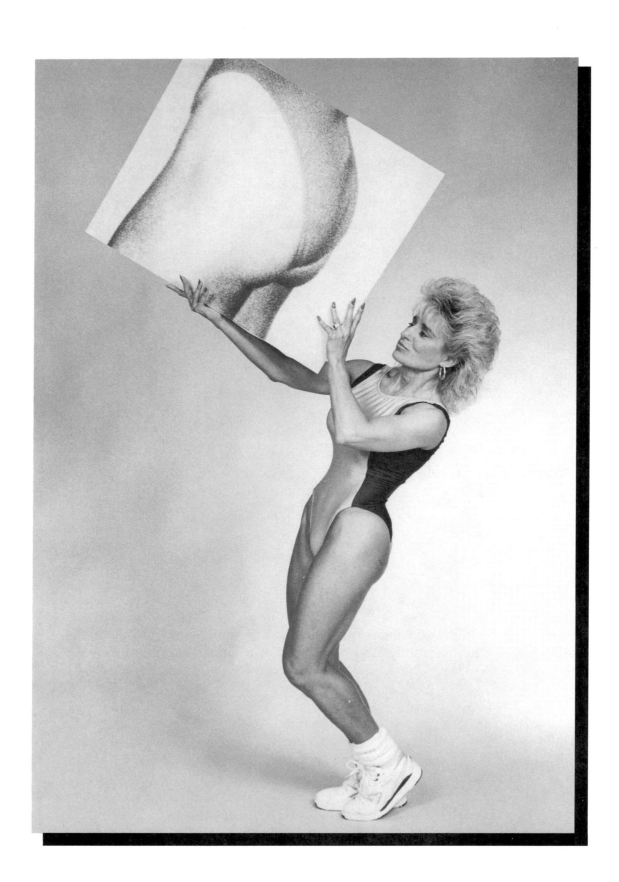

1

BOTTOMS UP!

Let's face it, ladies. When it comes to working out, it's time we put the emphasis where it's needed—on the bottom up. Most women carry the majority of their problem weight and cellulite in the thighs, the hips, the buttocks, and the stomach. In fact, most of us women are likely to have not only the proverbial pear shape, but also the apple-shaped stomach that plagues so many men. In other words, if the truth be told, we are stuck with BIG PROBLEMS from the waist down.

That's why I've written *Bottoms Up!* Not to eliminate upper-body work completely, but to provide a workout that will attack the problem of the lower and middle body head on, while at the same time giving due attention to the upper body. It's a workout that will once and for all solve the problem of big—or even thin but saggy—cellulite-ridden thighs, oversized saddle-bag hips, dimpled and descending buttocks, and fat rolls on the stomach that cause a woman to look pregnant twelve months of the year, even though she isn't expecting anything but more fat and cellulite unless she does something to turn things around.

I wrote this workout for myself as much as I wrote it for you. It happened quite naturally. You see, some time ago, I noticed that doing the same amount of exercise for the lower, middle, and upper body left me with a gorgeous upper body but a not-so-gorgeous lower and middle

1

body. I realized that in order to conquer those areas and make them look as good as my upper body, I had to add more exercises. I did this, and in time I achieved what is for me a perfect middle and lower body. (I'll never have narrow hips or tiny buttocks, but I've achieved the perfect look for my body shape.)

That's when I realized that all of my books tell women to do the same amount of work for all body parts—only suggesting that if they need extra work in certain areas, they follow a "go the extra mile" plan. In the meantime, I realized that I had always required myself to go the extra mile for my lower and middle body. I knew then that I could no longer give women an option. I had to ask them to do what I did—to "bomb away" at the lower and middle body so that they too could achieve their perfectly balanced body.

Bottoms Up! provides a fat-burning, muscle-shaping program that will create the total body of your dreams. It asks you to do the greatest number of exercises for your lower body (your thighs and hips/buttocks), where it is most needed; somewhat fewer exercises, but still a substantial number, for your middle body (your stomach); and the least amount of exercises (but enough to be tight, toned, and defined) for your upper body.

THE 7-5-3 PLAN

In other words, *Bottoms Up!* puts the emphasis where it's needed—on the bottom up. Its 7-5-3 plan, in ascending order, asks you to perform carefully paired exercises for each of the nine body parts: seven for your lower body (thighs and hip/butt area), five for your middle body (stomach area), and three for your upper body (chest, shoulders, biceps, triceps, and back areas) with "Wild Woman" and "Terminator" programs included for those women who also want to put greater emphasis on their upper bodies.

And I haven't even told you the best part yet. Now, for the first time in your life, you will no longer dread working out, because I have invented a new method of exercising that eliminates muscle fatigue yet allows you to work nonstop! Not only will the lower and middle body workout become a breeze, but the upper body workout will seem to go so much faster because all monotony will be gone. How can all of this be possible?

THE SECRET OF THIS WORKOUT

Bottoms Up! is based upon a new system of working out, one that I've developed by studying the techniques of champion bodybuilders. For years I've observed bodybuilders as they exercised body parts in pairs—a technique they call the "superset." Bodybuilders, however, use the term *superset* to mean the pairing of two exercises for the same body part, as well as the pairing of two exercises for different body parts. In other words, bodybuilders use one term, *superset*, to describe two different methods of working out. Although this overlap doesn't seem to bother bodybuilders (why should it? they spend most of their time working out and have ample opportunity to clarify whatever confusions they may have), it bothers me—because I know that the majority of my readers are not bodybuilders, and I don't want them to become confused. So I have coined a special term to describe the specific method of pairing that we will be using: *the interset.*

Simply explained, the interset is a method of exercising two *different* but compatible body parts in pairs. For example, you do one exercise for your thighs—and without resting, you do a companion exercise for your hip/buttock area. This is an interset. After each interset you are allowed a short rest, but you may choose not to take it, because you've already rested your nonworking muscle while you were exercising another muscle.

With the interset method of working out, when it comes time to do your second set, you don't dread it but are in fact ready to go. You never feel exhausted, no matter which body part you are exercising. You end up working nonstop without getting tired or overtraining a muscle (working so hard on a muscle that you wear it down rather than build it up), and in the bargain you can burn even more fat than you burned while using the program I developed for *The Fat-Burning Workout!*

Why? Because with the Fat-Burning Workout, you were doing three to five sets of various exercises for one body part before resting, and then going right back to that same body part for another three to five sets of the same exercise. That routine forced you to rest, or your muscles would have become fatigued. Not so with *Bottoms Up!* Since you are exercising different body parts in pairs, you can, if you choose, eliminate the rests altogether. Your muscles would not become fatigued, and because you would not be taking time at all between sets, you would of course burn that much more fat.

TWENTY-FOUR WORKOUT HOURS TO THE BODY OF YOUR DREAMS

In just twenty-four workout hours (twelve weeks of weight training, four to six days a week at twenty to thirty minutes per session), you will see your thighs, hips, buttocks, and stomach becoming tight, toned, cellulite free, and defined. Depending upon how out of shape and/or overweight you are, you may have reached your perfect body at that point. If not, you will have to work a little longer—perhaps another six months. But one thing is for sure. If you do not give up, if you keep on going, in a year's time you will have the body you dared only fantasize about. And just in case you need a little pep talk along the way, you can write to me at my P.O. box, and if you include a SASE, I'll personally answer your letter.

"Wait a minute," you may be thinking. "How come *The Fat-Burning Workout* says that we will go from fat to firm in only twenty-four days—and that we will reach our goal in six weeks?"

Since writing that book, I have come to realize that for many women it is really only the upper body that can get into perfect shape that quickly. The middle and lower body usually need a lot more work and a little more time.

THE FACTS ABOUT CELLULITE

Myth: Cellulite is genetic—you can't get rid of it.
Fact: Cellulite is stubborn, bunched-up fat—it will gradually disappear as you follow the Bottoms Up! Plan!

While it is true that some people are more genetically inclined to cellulite than others, everyone can get rid of it—and this means *you.*

The best proof to any claim are living examples. I am one of them. When I was thirty, my thighs and buttocks were already quite dimply with developing cellulite, and by the time I was in my midthirties, those areas resembled a cross between an orange peel and cheesecake. (Cellulite is formed by enlarged fat cells that join together and attach themselves to connecting fibrous tissue just beneath the surface of the skin, giving the skin a bumpy, craterlike appearance.)

I hated to look in the mirror. That's when I began my desperate search.

I discovered that creams, gels, and wraps of all kinds were useless. All they did was give a one-day respite from some of the deeper craters of cellulite. In a day or two, the cellulite would return to its original form.

Finally, I discovered weight training, aerobic exercise, and a low-fat eating plan, and I combined these elements into a system that gets rid of cellulite once and for all. Now, with time and persistence, *anyone*, no matter how bad their condition, can do it.

I've put hundreds of women on the program, and they too now testify to the amazing changes that have taken place in their bodies. They range in age from eighteen (yes, believe it or not, some women begin to get cellulite at that age—and younger) to well into their sixties, and older. And some of these women are not really overweight. They're what I call a "skinny fat": they are out of shape, they have little or no muscle tone, and the small amount of fat they do have lies bunched up just beneath the skin, forming orange-peel cellulite!

How do you get rid of cellulite? There's really no mystery about it. As you perform the weight-training exercises prescribed in this book, and at the same time follow the low-fat eating plan, two things happen:

1. Muscle begins to form in the cellulite-ridden areas.
2. Fat in these areas (and all over your body, too) begins to burn up and disappear.

Because they are also aerobic in nature, the exercises, in addition to building muscle, help you to burn away that much more bunched-up fat, or cellulite.

As you continue to work out and consume a low-fat diet, in time your previously dimpled, cellulite-ridden body parts inevitably become smooth and firm, defined and shapely. Cellulite has been replaced by firm muscle.

Diet alone won't do it. Exercise alone won't do it. Diet and haphazard exercise won't do it. It's the special formula of diet and the right combination of exercise that gets results.

YOU CAN DO IT AT HOME WITH VERY LITTLE EQUIPMENT

The beauty of this program is that you can do it in your home with very little equipment—for a fraction of the price it would cost you to join a gym or fitness center. All you need are three sets of light dumbbells and a bench. And if you don't have a bench, you can do those exercises that require a bench at the edge of a bed, chair, or sofa—and on the floor.

Working out at home is a pleasure for those of us who want to save not only money, but time and perhaps embarrassment, too. Some days the very thought of making the effort of going to and from a fitness center and of having to deal with others looking on as we sweat and groan is enough to make us forget the whole thing.

If you do want to join a gym or fitness center, of course you can do the workout there—either with the dumbbells provided by the management or, following "Gym Workout" instructions that I provide, with the machines.

WHAT YOU CAN EXPECT FROM THIS PROGRAM

If you commit yourself to the program, here's what you can expect to get from it:

- A reduced dress or pants size in a matter of weeks
- The steady loss of fat weight (not muscle or water) at the rate of one-quarter pound to two pounds a week (depending upon how over-weight you are now) until you achieve your ideal body
- Cellulite-free thighs, hips, buttocks, and stomach in approximately twenty-four workout hours if you are not more than thirty pounds overweight, or the same in six months to a year no matter how fat or out of shape you are!
- Feminine muscularity and definition in all the right places in a matter of months
- The workout habit for life
- A "never be bored" lifetime fitness maintenance plan
- An increased rate of metabolism because you have added muscle to your body composition, so that you will not have to diet as much to maintain your weight
- A "never be hungry" accelerated fat-loss plan
- Increased energy
- Improved posture
- Increased self-confidence
- A healthier heart and greater lung capacity

HOW MANY MINUTES A DAY?

All of this will be accomplished in twenty to thirty minutes a day, depending upon how fast you work and whether or not you take advantage of your allowed rests. Did I say "a day"? Excuse me. I mean four days a week of weight training. But then again, I really do mean every day, because I don't want you to lie stagnant on the other days. On the three days you are not weight training, I will encourage you to perform an aerobic activity of your choice. Although *Bottoms Up!* is, in and of itself, an aerobic workout (you keep your heart rate in the ideal fat-burning range as you work), I want you to include your favorite aerobic activities as well, to round out the program and to further increase your heart and lung capacity. I also don't want you to get lazy on those days off.

So if at all possible, no days off. It's better that way. And it's easier to establish a routine that way. You don't take days off from brushing your teeth, do you? It's a habit. This too will soon become a habit. A mere twenty to thirty minutes a day for life—and I do mean, for *your* life. (Aerobic choices will be further discussed in chapters 7 and 8.)

Before I say another word, I want to get a few things straight. I want to talk about muscles—why women need them, indeed, must have them—and to explain how working with weights actually solves the problem of thinning bones (osteoporosis). I also want to tell you why medical doctors, sports physiologists, and fitness experts are now in general agreement that there's no way to get in perfect shape—health and body shape—unless you work out with weights. Finally, I want to reassure you that you will be allowed to eat plenty of food while you're losing your fat.

MUSCLES, MUSCLES, MUSCLES: DO WOMEN *REALLY* NEED THEM?

Yes. Yes. Yes. Emphatically yes—for five very important reasons.

Look Thinner

Muscle makes you look and feel thinner. It's true! Muscle takes up less space than fat does, so pound for pound, if you have more muscle than another woman who weighs the same as you, you can be at least two dress sizes smaller. And this will be the case even though your muscles are small and petite—not the "Arnold" kind!

Eat More Without Getting Fat

Muscles allow you to eat more food without getting fat because muscle is the only body material that is active. Muscle actually "scintillates" (the muscle fibers vibrate ever so slightly, rather than lie stagnant), and it does so twenty-four hours a day—even when you're sitting in a chair or sleeping in your bed. (Bone and fat just "sit there" and vegetate.)

The fact is, once you put muscle on your body, you will burn an additional 20 to 30 calories an hour! Just think of the dieting you won't have to do for those 480 to 600 calories a day! And I'm talking about the moderate muscles you will get by using this program. (Hulks such as champion bodybuilders actually burn 50 to 75 additional calories per hour. In fact, that's why they eat so much more than the average person. If they didn't, they'd starve!)

That muscle allows you to eat more can be seen in the way, comparatively speaking, men get away with murder in the food department. Pound for pound, men have always been able to eat more than women without getting fat. Years ago, before nutritional research, we had no idea why this was so. Now we know that because men naturally have more muscle than women (their bodies just make muscle more readily because of their naturally higher level of testosterone, a muscle-building hormone), they burn more fat.

Now that we know the secret, it's time to start getting some muscles! Why should the men have all the perks?

Beat the Aging Process
(Look at Me—I'm Pushing Fifty)

Did you know that muscle makes your body "youthe" as you age? Let me explain. Every year after the age of thirty, muscles atrophy a small amount. No one knows exactly how much, but experts say it is about 5 percent a year. If you do nothing to prevent this normal muscle attrition, by the time you are forty, your body shape will have significantly changed. Let's use a typical male as an example. Perhaps he was moderately athletic in college and, in fact, was quite well built and muscular, but not bulky. He looked great the last time you saw him, at the age of twenty-nine, although he had not participated in sports since college and had rarely worked out since that time.

You lose touch with him but happen to run into him ten years later. He is now nearing forty, and although he still wears the same size pants and shirt—something has changed. Instead of looking like the sexy, athletic man you knew, he now appears a bit "middle-aged." What could it be? He still has a head of thick black curly hair. His face hasn't changed much—not that you can notice. Now you see it. It's his body shape. His shoulders are very slightly stooped, his arms are thinner. His legs are not as hard, and he has a growing paunch where a "washboard" stomach used to be. His posture has changed. He doesn't throw his shoulders back as far. And the stride is gone. Now he merely plods along. Will that walk soon become a shuffle? What's wrong? He is not fat.

The answer is clear. The poor fellow is simply the victim of time—muscle attrition, and all the dieting in the world can't help him (he may foolishly think that all he has to do is diet and get rid of that little paunch, and then he will look like his old self again). The only thing that could help this man is appropriate training with weights. He doesn't have to accept his lot. And neither do women!

I talked about men first, because the loss of muscle is most noticeable in the male gender—for two reasons: women don't usually have as much muscular development as men to begin with, and women often get fatter than men, and then become obsessed with losing that fat. They don't realize that they have a double problem—muscle atrophy *and* weight gain, and they deal with only the weight gain.

Most women don't realize that their muscles have begun to atrophy, because the excess fat covers the thinning muscles with thick layers of cushioning. Such women don't discover their muscle loss until they shed the excess fat. That's when they get the big disappointing surprise. After all the weight is gone, they look in the mirror expecting to see the shapely, youthful body they had ten years ago, but instead, to their horror, they see a thin but drastically changed physique. They see thighs that drape over kneecaps, buttocks that sag, a lower stomach that still protrudes (no girdle of muscle to hold it in), and arms that are spongey and soft.

That's when these women either give up and get fat again, or are fortunate enough to find a fitness regimen that will get them into shape. But they could have accomplished two things at a time, had they worked out with weights while they were dieting! They could have lost the weight and at the same time tightened, toned, defined, and shaped the muscles under the fat. Then when that last pound of fat was gone, *voilà*, their dream body would have been already there.

Once a woman starts working out, whether it be while she is still fat or after she has lost the fat, the muscles begin to grow and develop—in effect, to youthe rather than continue to atrophy and age. How does this happen?

By working with weights, you put back the muscle that you lost every year after thirty—and then some. By putting back and then building more muscle than you previously had, you make your actual body composition younger than it was in your twenties. I did it. Look at the photograph of me at twenty-four, a year after marriage. I had gone from 98 pounds to 115 pounds, and had already begun to appear matronly. I was too ashamed to be seen in a bathing suit. And look at me now. I lost fat and gained muscle weight. Now I weigh the same 115 pounds (see my "After" photo), but look at the difference. (None of my pictures are touched up. What you see is the real me!) If I didn't work out with weights, I would be "hanging" everywhere, and my body would be covered with cellulite (bunched-up fat). I would also be much fatter! (I continued to gain weight until I began working out.)

Be Strong and Independent

Fourth, muscle gives you strength, and with it, independence and confidence. Aren't you sick and tired of being at the mercy of men to carry packages, open jars, and open heavy doors? Please don't misunderstand me. I'm very traditional in many ways. If a man is within ten feet of me and if he's willing, I am delighted to let him carry my heavy package, open that difficult jar, and wrestle with that heavy door. But what if there is no man in sight, or what if I don't feel like dealing with that particular man, or what if I'm in a hurry. I like the feeling of being able to say, "I can handle it. I don't have to wait for a man."

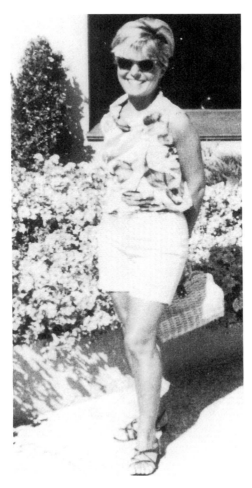

Joyce Vedral—24, 115 lbs. without muscle

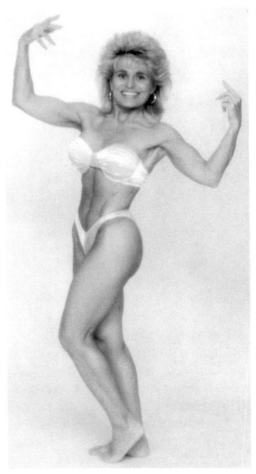

Joyce Vedral—49, 115 lbs. with muscle

Wow! Muscle Is Sexy!

Finally, muscle is sexy. Very sexy. It makes you feel sensual and sleek. It gives your body near-perfect symmetry. It puts curves and definition in all the right places. It is exciting to the touch—firm and toned rather than soft and mushy. Women love to see and feel the muscle on their own bodies—and men love it, too. In fact, men go wild when they see or touch a femininely muscular woman. (I must emphasize that I am not talking about the competitive bodybuilding women who work out three hours a day with heavy weights and appear to be men with a woman's head pasted on!) Believe me, you won't get more muscles than I have if you follow this program.

So it is clear that women need muscles—just the right kind of muscles, petite shapely muscles in all the right places. And that is what you'll get with this program! I personally guarantee it.

BONES, BONES, BONES: AN INSURANCE POLICY FOR THE FUTURE, AND A REMEDY FOR THE PRESENT!

Who cares about bones anyway? I know I never did. But with all the talk about women over thirty losing bone tissue to the point of danger, and then with the recent proof that working with weights increases bone density and indeed reverses osteoporosis, I do now.

If you work consistently with this program, you will never have a problem with thinning bones! You see, when you work with weights, you're not only putting stress on the muscle, you're putting stress on the bone as well, and you're making the bone stronger and thicker as you make the muscle stronger and bigger.

But what if you already have a problem with thinning bones and are in the beginning stages of osteoporosis. There is wonderful news. The proof is in. Working out with weights actually reverses osteoporosis. Dr. Sydney Bonnick, director of Osteoporosis Services at the Cooper Clinic in Dallas, Texas, can cite case after case of people who have literally reversed osteoporosis by working with weights. He talks about one woman who had experienced early bone decay—she was only forty-one. But after ten months of working with weights, her bone mass increased by 2.5 percent. But I'm not as impressed with a forty-one-year-old's progress as I am with the eighty- and ninety-year-olds who were previously unable to walk without a cane, climb stairs, or indeed, pick themselves up from the floor if they fell. (Previously, their muscles and bones were too weak to assist them in getting up, and they had to wait in the hope that someone would come along and discover that they had fallen.) As a result of working out with weights, now these senior citizens can do things that they had thought they could never do again!

The fact is, all the calcium supplements in the world cannot do for you what weight training can do. If you don't have a problem with thinning bones—great. Think of this workout as an insurance policy. If you do have a problem with thinning bones, this program will help to change all of that.

THE EXPERTS AGREE!

For the past forty years, fitness experts such as Joe Weider, Jack La Lanne, Dan Lurie, and others have been celebrating the virtues of working out with weights—for strength, health, and a beautiful body. But they were voices crying in the wilderness, because the large majority of experts emphasized only two aspects of fitness: diet and aerobics. It seemed as if in their eyes weight training didn't even exist. They chose to ignore it or to give it quick mention as a "sport."

For the past five years medical doctors and exercise physiologists have been exploring the benefits of weight training and have now come to realize that it is working out with weights, not aerobics or dieting, that can best improve muscle and bone strength and quality of life. In fact, Kenneth Cooper, the man who started everyone on aerobics, admits that aerobics are just not enough! His exercise facility at the Cooper Clinic has now undergone a total rearrangement of space to include room for weight-training equipment.

Weight training's "in" status with the medical and fitness experts of the world was signed, sealed, and delivered in 1991, when the American College of Sports Medicine altered its fitness guidelines—guidelines that had not been touched for twelve years—to include working out with weights. (They have always advocated aerobics, now they recommend both aerobics and weight training.)

Health and fitness institutions all over America are getting on board. In fact, the Pritikin Longevity Center, the renowned heart and health and fitness center, has asked me to help them set up a weight-training program. People who do aerobics only, such as jogging or stair climbing, have lower-body strength, but they don't have enough upper-body strength. They now know that they must add weight training to their fitness regimen to order to achieve balanced fitness.

I am now in the process of working with the Pritikin Longevity Center on a free-weight program for people who, on the average, range in age from fifty to eighty years old!

MORE THAN HEALTH AND FITNESS— A PERFECT BODY

If you want to achieve a near-perfect body shape in addition to the health benefits discussed above, it isn't enough to follow a plan proposed by those who know just enough about weight training to improve your health. You must follow the plan of those who also know how to reshape the body—the plan of bodybuilders, the plan contained in this book.

Now don't become alarmed. You will not get as big as a bodybuilder if you follow this program. You will simply achieve near-perfect symmetry but with much smaller muscles. You see, since you will be working with much lighter weights and exercising for much shorter time periods than do bodybuilders, you will get a "mini" body rather than a "hulky" body—but one that is perfectly shaped.

Go to the Expert!

Champion bodybuilders are experts in body shaping. It is their life. They know exactly how to create a perfectly shaped thigh, an ideal shoulder, high, tight buttocks, and so on. They spend all of their waking hours learning just how to do such things. Indeed, they make their living on how their bodies appear. If a bodybuilder goes into a contest, and her waist appears too large, she loses the contest. She knows exactly how to go back to the weights and make herself a smaller-looking waist. If her buttocks are too big, she knows exactly how to go back to the gym and make them high and tight. So it goes for every body part.

I have worked with champion bodybuilders for years, as a writer for *Muscle and Fitness* magazine. They have told me their secrets, and I have tried them on myself and others; I have modified them to work on men and women who don't want to look like bodybuilders but who want to have the perfect body.

So why go to people who know just a little about body shaping? If you have a foot problem, would you go to a general practitioner? Of course not. You would go to a podiatrist, a specialist in foot problems. If you had a neck strain, would you go to a general practitioner? Of course not. You'd go to a chiropractor or an orthopaedic surgeon. So why waste your time training with people who can only give you a little help. Why not go straight to the source where you can get the perfect body in the shortest possible time.

I am the expert. I have spent years perfecting bodybuilding principles and tailoring them to the average woman or man who wants a perfectly shaped body.

OTHER BENEFITS OF WORKING OUT WITH WEIGHTS

Working out with weights as described in this book will do more for you than give you shapely muscles and strong bones. It will decrease your chance of injury if you are a participant in any sport. Most sports injuries are "musculoskeletal" (involving the muscles and/or the bones).

Whether you play tennis, raquetball, squash, or golf, or any other sport for that matter, this workout will help to insure against injury because it will strengthen your joints and eliminate the muscle weakness and imbalance that causes such injuries. It will also increase your stamina and power in that sport. Your arms will be stronger and will be able to swing at the ball that much harder—making it go that much farther. Your legs will be that much stronger and will be able to run that much faster without becoming exhausted.

If you suffer from back, neck, or shoulder pain, this program can work wonders. Because you will be exercising every major muscle group (nine body parts), you will create a balanced posture that will help to eliminate back, neck, and shoulder pain. Your back will be especially helped by the stomach workout (it is abdominal muscles that help to support the back).

WILL YOU HAVE TO GIVE UP EATING?

Absolutely not! In fact, the Bottoms Up! Eating Plan allows you to eat more filling food than ever before. Recent nutritional discoveries have enabled me to create a much-improved diet that will help you to lose your excess body fat faster than ever before. You will be allowed plenty to eat—whenever you are hungry—and it won't be grass or lettuce leaves you're allowed. You'll get to eat plenty of potatoes, even sweet potatoes, and more whole-grain pasta, brown rice, and hot cereals than you could expect to eat on any diet—and still lose fat galore. You'll hear all about the new eating plan in chapter 9. In the meantime, rest assured—there's nothing to dread. You won't starve while you're shedding the fat.

But there is something to look forward to. Once you reach your goal, you will be allowed to indulge in any and every food you crave one day a week.

THE PERFECTLY BALANCED PROGRAM

After all is said and done, the ideal fitness regimen includes a weight-training program that will strengthen and develop the muscles and bones and shape the body into its most perfect form; an aerobic program that will increase heart and lung capacity; and a well-balanced nutritional program that will never allow an individual to go hungry, while at the same time decreasing excess body fat until the ideal range is achieved. This program includes all three.

In the past, people have chosen diet as the only way to fitness. Then people became aware of the benefits of aerobics, and they added that activity to dieting, hoping to get in shape. Now, finally, weight training has been recognized as the missing link. Perhaps that is what has been preventing you from getting into shape up till now.

IT DOESN'T MATTER HOW FAT YOU ARE— EVEN A HUNDRED POUNDS OR MORE OVERWEIGHT

In closing this chapter, I must speak to those ladies who may be fifty, seventy-five, or a hundred or more pounds overweight. This program is for you, too. It is most important that you *not wait* until you have lost the weight before you start working out. By following this workout, you will increase your weight loss and, at the same time, build a firm body that will be formed under your fat and revealed once the fat is gone. Don't worry. This workout will *not* make you look *bigger*.

Don't make the mistake of thinking that it's better to first diet until all the fat is gone, and then start working out. If you do this, you will sell yourself short on two counts. You'll lose out on the fat-burning power of muscle, and you'll be depressed rather than thrilled when you reach your weight goal, only to see that your skinny body—the one that you suffered for—is sagging and flabby. Wouldn't it be better to kill two birds with one stone and start the workout at the same time as the diet?

In summary, no matter what you do, don't say to yourself, "I'm too fat. This program is not for me." Sure. It will take you a little longer to get in shape (see chapter 2), but so what. At least you will be on the right track!

Notes:
Page 12: Interview with Dr. Sydney Bonnick, director, Osteoporosis Services, Cooper Clinic, Dallas, Texas, by John Stossel, ABC News. *20/20*, May 10, 1991, show #1119. New York: Journal Graphics, pp. 7–9.

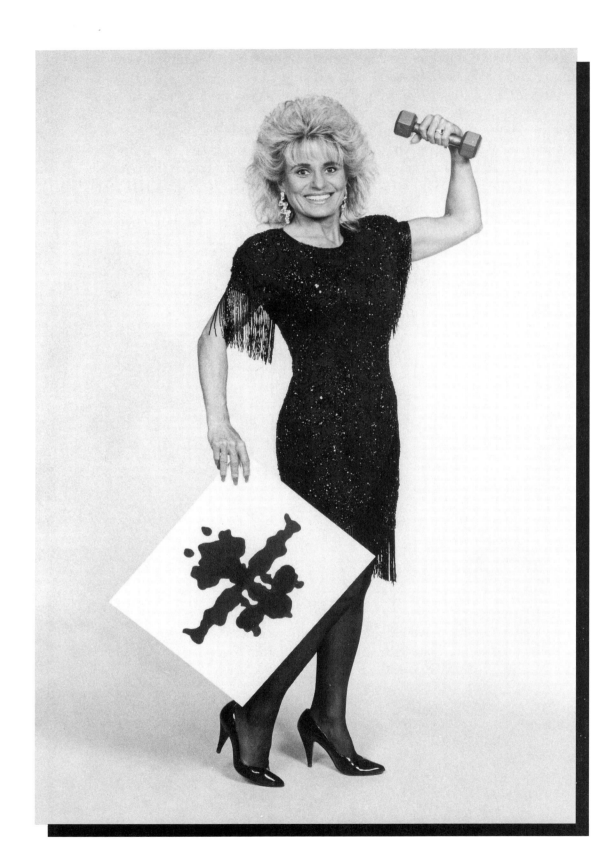

2

WHAT TO EXPECT— PHYSICALLY AND PSYCHOLOGICALLY

As you perform the Bottoms Up! Workout, certain things will happen to your body—and your mind. What will happen to your body and how fast it will happen depend upon the shape you are in now. What will happen to your mind will depend upon your psychological makeup.

The following chapter is meant to help you prepare for what is ahead. It is meant to give you a realistic picture of how fast you will lose weight and see firm, well-defined muscle take the place of fat, and to explain why at times nothing will seem to be happening—and then suddenly, a clear burst of progress.

It is also crucial to have advance knowledge of the mental aspect of the workout. A basic understanding of the way the mind works when it comes to self-discipline can head off trouble for you and, in fact, ensure that you make it through this time. By reading the psychological portion of this chapter, you can learn about the tricks your mind will try to play, and be prepared for—and indeed, avoid—the traps and save your workout! Indeed, by the time you finish reading this chapter, you will know that if you want to do it, you *can* work out and get in shape, no matter what happens—and you will feel in control of your life in a way that you never did before.

First let's talk about exactly what will happen to your body as you begin and then continue to work out. Then we'll discuss ways to make sure that your mind is in full cooperation with your body so that your success will be guaranteed.

ONE TO TEN POUNDS OVERWEIGHT

You are in the most difficult category when it comes to weight loss. Your body is quite pleased with its extra poundage and, in fact, is planning to keep that fat around, just in case there is a future famine. You see, the body is not aware that we are no longer in the era of the caveman, and is still concerned about food availability. Therefore, the body will make every effort to retain up to seven pounds of additional fat and will be in no hurry to get rid of even ten pounds of fat—"just in case."

What's so terrible about being ten pounds overweight? Actually, you are not "fat." For health purposes nothing is so terrible about it. Indeed, most height-weight charts (see page 32) allow about a ten-pound range, but most of us consider ourselves overweight if we are on the higher end of the range. So what is so terrible? It is that we are "so near and yet so far." We don't want to be ten pounds overweight. If we had our own way, we'd rather be five or ten pounds underweight, because we feel just the way the body's survival system feels, only in reverse: we would like a reserve of "thinness" just in case we get depressed and begin an eating binge.

What is the answer to the dilemma? The first thing you must understand is that when you are only ten pounds overweight, you will lose weight at a very slow rate, and the closer to the lower end of the scale you are, the harder it will be to lose weight. For example, if you are only one or two pounds overweight, it can seem like it takes forever to get rid of those pounds.

In order to lose those last ten pounds, you must resign yourself to the fact that it's going to take time. Sure. You can do it quickly by going on a crash diet and starving the fat off your body, but in the end you will be fatter than when you started out. That's because once you reach your weight goal, the moment you are off guard, your body will sabotage you and eat everything in sight until it replaces the lost fat—and then some. The only way to get rid of the last ten pounds (and any weight, for that matter, even if you are a hundred pounds overweight) is to do it by feeding the body a nutritious low-fat diet that will result in a slow, steady weight loss.

How slowly will the body give up its extra fat if you are only up to ten pounds overweight? For the first three pounds you may lose an average of a pound a week. Then you may slow down to a half or three-quarters of a pound a week for the next three pounds. You may lose your last four pounds at an average of a quarter to a half pound a week, and if you have any lapses in your diet or training, you will lose it even more slowly. (You may lose it more slowly anyway, depending upon how stubborn your body is about giving up those last few pounds.)

There's another important point to remember. There will be some weeks when you don't lose any weight at all. Some weeks the scale may even show a weight gain. There are three reasons for this. The body loses weight over time on an "average" weekly weight loss. It does not monitor itself to lose exactly, say, half a pound a week. Some weeks you will lose nothing. Then suddenly, the scale will drop by two or three pounds. If you lose nothing or even gain on those weeks when you know you are doing everything right, it will be tempting to give up and go on an eating binge. If you realize that weight fluctuation is normal, however, and continue to work out and follow the diet, the scale will move downward in time.

But what about the other two factors that contribute to the strange behavior of the scale even though you are dieting, behavior that makes the scale stay the same for weeks or even go up before it goes down? They are muscle and water. Let's take muscle first.

Muscle Weighs More Than Fat but Takes Up Less Space

In order to get into shape, as you know, it is not enough to simply lose weight. You must also tone up. But what does that mean? It means putting small, shapely muscles all over your body while at the same time losing excess body fat, so that your body no longer feels soft and flabby to the touch, but firm, instead.

When you are working out with weights, even the light weights described in this program, and are following the low-fat diet, you will be losing fat and gaining muscle, and your body composition will be slowly changing. In as little as three weeks' time, your body will have given up, say, two and a half pounds of fat, but at the same time, you may have gained a half a pound of muscle (more or less, depending upon how fast your body builds muscle). So what you will see on the scale after three weeks of diligent attention to your diet and the workout may be a weight loss of only two pounds.

Wait. Don't throw this book across the room. This is actually good news. It's what you want. You see, as you lose fat and gain muscle, your body gets smaller! You fit into a smaller size in jeans and a dress, but often, the scale goes down little or nothing! How can this be? You see, muscle takes up less space than fat but weighs more. In three months (or less) you will have lost ten pounds of fat—that fluffy stuff that is like a pillow of feathers and takes up so much space—but at the same time you may have put on two pounds of muscle, which is like lead, taking up little space but weighing more than fat. So your scale weight shows only a eight-pound weight loss, and you are frustrated and say to yourself, "I'm still three pounds overweight." But you are not overweight. In fact, if you look in the mirror, you are leaner and more in shape than ever before in your life, and you are wearing the smallest size jeans you've ever worn. But you are still operating on the idea of having a light, fluffy, fatty body, and your "scale" standard is based upon the antiquated idea that you are made of more fat than muscle.

What? So you're not going to work with weights if it's going to mean that you won't lose weight on the scale as fast as possible? This would be the biggest mistake you could make, because as you know, what you need is muscle in order to be tight, toned, shapely, and well defined. The mirror tells the true story, not the scale. There is no choice in the matter. And as discussed before, muscle also allows you to eat more without getting fat. It's just a matter of educating yourself and readjusting your thinking. In fact, if I had my way, you'd throw the scale out the window and make the mirror your new scale. But for those of you who won't do that, I've provided you with a new way to look at weight charts (see page 32).

In addition, there is yet another factor to consider when you are vigilantly watching the scale and trying to lose weight. That is water fluctuation.

Water-Weight Fluctuation

Our body's water retention varies from day to day and from week to week. If you happen to eat foods high in sodium one day, the next day your body could retain up to three pounds of excess water. If you eat high-sodium foods for a few days in a row, your body may retain up to five or six pounds of excess water. It can get even worse. If you take strong prescription water-elimination pills for a few days and drop your water to extremely low levels, when you stop taking the pills, you may gain up to ten pounds of water in a matter of three days as your body tries to revive itself by "sucking up" as much water as it can and retaining it. (I know this because it happened to me.)

Why am I telling you all of this? The fact is that water weight varies, and it can drive you out of your mind. When you're trying to lose those last few pounds, the best thing you can do is to keep your sodium at a normal level (see page 248). Enjoy your life. Don't cut your sodium to practically zero and fool yourself into believing you have lost fat weight when in reality your body is dehydrated. On the other hand, don't eat pickles, canned foods, and other high-sodium delights, or you may well feel bloated and get discouraged when the scale shows a weight gain rather than a weight loss, even though you've been an angel, keeping to the low-fat diet and working out exactly the way you're supposed to.

If you keep your sodium intake at a moderate level—and if you realize that even so, there will be days when your overall sodium consumption is greater than others and that your body can retain a pound or two of water on occasion—you won't panic when the scale shows a temporary weight gain. (If you followed my advice and refused to get on the scale, you would save yourself all of this anxiety, but in case you don't, forewarned is forearmed. You can save yourself from giving up if at least you know what's happening.)

There is yet another reason for water retention, and that is menstruation. As you know, women typically retain up to five pounds of water around the time of their period, and they lose that water a few days after their period ends. It is foolish to take water pills (unless, of course, the water retention gives you headaches or in other ways makes you physically uncomfortable, and your doctor prescribes the pills). After all, if your body is retaining water around the time of your menstruation, it does so for a reason. Apparently your body needs that water for a short time. My theory is and always has been "Don't fool with Mother Nature." Just live with it and let it pass. Tell yourself, "Oh, well. I've had my period. This water weight will be gone in a few days."

I've had to do television shows while retaining five pounds of water, and lately, having learned the hard way, I've refused to take a water pill. No one notices the extra bloat because the muscles take attention away from any faults. If you follow the Bottoms Up! Plan, you'll soon be in the same position. You'll never be thrilled about water retention, but it won't bother you nearly as much as it does now, when you're not in shape.

In summary, then, when it comes to losing weight and you are only ten pounds or less overweight, you must realize that the body gives up fat slowly because of the survival system, that muscle weighs more than fat, and that water retention shifts according to sodium consumption and the menstrual cycle. The best favor you can do yourself is to refuse to get on the scale for a month at a time and just look in the mirror. But what will you see in the mirror?

What You Will See and Feel

In three weeks or less of doing my workout, you will begin to see pretty lines of definition beginning to form in your shoulder and upper back area. Your biceps will begin to feel firmer and will indeed show the beginnings of a real curve when you "make a muscle." Your triceps will still appear loose, but they will feel tighter to the touch. You may see some definition in your upper chest and some "cleavage" beginning to be formed between your breasts. Your stomach will feel tighter, and if you flex your abdominal muscles, you may see a line or two of definition in your side abdominals (oblique muscles) and even some slight definition in your upper abdominals. That little pot on your lower abdominal area will be the last to go, and your thighs and buttocks will take a little more work.

In six weeks, more definition will be popping up everywhere. Your chest muscles will continue to form, and your breasts will begin to appear uplifted. Your triceps muscle will be firm and need only a little more work. Your lower belly's pot will be significantly reduced but, depending upon childbirth and years of neglect, may take much longer to go away. As you continue to work, you will build a steel girdle of muscles that will hold that pot in. It may take six months to a year before your lower belly is absolutely perfect, but you'll see continual improvement along the way. Your thighs and buttocks will begin to feel tighter, your thighs will show definition on the inner area, and your buttocks will be markedly lifted.

In three months your entire body will be firmer to the touch. Your shoulders, chest, arms, and back will be well defined. Your triceps will be firm to the touch and will no longer jiggle. Your abdominal muscles will be well defined, and the lower pot will be nearly or completely gone. Your thighs will be firm and have clear definition, and you will notice a muscle (quadriceps) has been formed in the front area. Your buttocks will be significantly lifted. Some people will say you are perfect—and at times you will think, "Hmm. Maybe I am." But you will still feel as if there is more improvement to be attained—and you are right.

In six months your body will be harder—sexier. Your muscles will begin to become "seasoned" as you begin to make them a natural part of yourself. Any stubborn, lagging body parts will begin to "get with the program." Your triceps will be firm and toned and well defined. They will no longer wave in the wind like a flag when you raise your arms. Your stomach will continue to improve until the pot is completely gone. Your thighs will give up any last bit of cellulite. Your buttocks will be high, firm, and well shaped. Are you perfect? Perhaps. Some will be. But others may take longer.

You may look at your thighs and still not be happy. You may notice that the skin is still hanging ever so slightly near the kneecap. This may be true if you are over forty. You may decide to put a larger muscle there to eliminate that problem (see page 81). After six months you will specialize, modifying parts of the program in order to zone in on any unperfected body part.

You will keep going with this "zoning in" until in a year's time you are absolutely perfect—even in your own eyes. But believe it or not, year by year, as you continue to work out and to switch between the various maintenance plans, you will continue to see improvement!

ELEVEN TO TWENTY-FIVE POUNDS OVERWEIGHT

If you are in this category, you will lose weight a little faster than the people in the above category. How much faster depends upon where you are on the scale. If you are closer to twenty-five pounds overweight, you will lose weight faster. If you are closer to only eleven pounds overweight, you will lose weight more slowly. The bottom line is, the heavier you are, the faster you lose, because your body's survival system will cooperate with you rather than fight you. (The caveman's body knew that if it was overweight it would not be able to run from wild animals.)

If you are on the higher end of the scale, you will lose up to an average of a pound to a pound and a half a week, until you are only ten pounds overweight. Then you may lose as those in the previous category. Keep in mind that at times the scale will move more slowly, because you are making muscles that weigh more than fat but take up less space. Your pant size may go down sooner than your scale weight! But so what. Do you carry the scale around and say, "But look at my weight"? Of course not. You carry that butt around, and people see it getting smaller! Water weight fluctuation may also frustrate you, so don't become preoccupied with the scale. Instead, look in the mirror. (Please read "Muscle Weighs

More Than Fat..." and "Water-Weight Fluctuation" on pages 21–23. This is very important.)

What You Will See and Feel

In three weeks you will see pretty lines of definition beginning to form in your upper back and shoulder area. Your biceps may show a definite curve when you make a muscle, and you will feel your triceps beginning to tighten. Your chest will begin to show some definition. Your stomach, thighs, and buttocks will still seem fat, although when you touch them, they will feel tighter.

In six weeks you will continue to gain definition, and your entire body will feel and look tighter. Your biceps muscle will continue to become firm and round, your triceps will not be as jiggly, and more cleavage will appear between your breasts. Your stomach size will have gone down significantly, and you will begin to see definition in your side abdominal (oblique) muscles and a trace of definition in your upper abdominal area. Your thighs will begin to show change as definition begins to appear in your inner thigh and cellulite is reduced. Your buttocks will begin to be lifted.

In three months you will be nearly at your weight goal, and definition will be popping up everywhere. Your triceps will be firm—and getting firmer all the time—and your breasts will be significantly lifted. Your biceps muscle will be hard and sensual. Your thighs will be toned and have a shapely muscle with inner thigh definition. Your buttocks will be going in the right direction—up—and they will look and feel firmer and more toned. Your abdominal area will show upper and side definition, but you may need a little more work on the lower pot.

In six months you will have achieved your goal, but as above, you will want to go another six months to get that "set" effect. (Read the discussions on results after six months and a year on page 24. They are the same for you).

TWENTY-SIX POUNDS TO FIFTY POUNDS OVERWEIGHT

If you are on the lower end of the scale, your body may follow the guidelines as above. You should really read both of the previous sections. If you are on the higher end of the scale, here's what you can expect: Since your body is clearly overweight, it will cooperate fully in weight loss. You can expect to lose an average of one and a half pounds a week. (Note that I say average; there will be weeks when you lose two or more pounds on the scale, and weeks when you lose only a pound or less, due to reasons discussed above. Read "Muscle Weighs More Than Fat..." and "Water-Weight Fluctuation" on pages 21–23.)

What You Will See and Feel

In three weeks you will begin to see definition in your upper back and shoulder area. Your biceps will begin to show a curve when you make a muscle, but your triceps will still feel soft to the touch because the developing muscle will still be covered with too much fat to show a change. You will show some definition in your upper chest area. Your stomach, thighs, and buttocks may feel slightly harder, but they will still be covered with too much fat to show any visible change.

In six weeks you will continue to see definition in the above areas. Your biceps will take shape and show hardness and curves. Your stomach will have gone down significantly. You will see a trace of definition in your inner thigh area and will feel a tightening there. Your buttocks will be slightly lifted, but you won't know whether it's your imagination or not.

In three months definition will continue. Your biceps will be clear and strong. Your triceps will be much tighter, but definition may not show if you are still overweight. Your stomach will have continued to reduce in size, and you will begin to see definition in your side and upper abdominal muscles. Your lower pot, however, will still be there, but it will be reduced in size. Your buttocks will clearly be lifted but may need more work. There will be a muscle (quadriceps) forming in your front thigh, and you will begin to see definition on your inner thigh.

In six months you will be at your goal—or almost there—depending upon how much overweight you are (see previous sections if you are not at your weight goal yet). Your body will be tight, toned, and well defined.

You may still need some work on stubborn areas (see the discussions on results after six months and a year on page 24).

MORE THAN FIFTY POUNDS OVERWEIGHT

More than fifty pounds overweight, more than a hundred pounds overweight! What? How can I group you all in the same category? I do this for two reasons:

1. The body will cooperate fully in weight loss if you are more than fifty pounds overweight. You will lose an average of one and a half to two pounds of fat a week.

2. Many of your developing muscles will be obscured by the fat until you get down to about forty pounds overweight, and then more and more muscles will begin to show up (see below).

I don't want you to be discouraged. Note that water retention may shift your weight from week to week, so the scale may not always show a significant drop. Muscle development may also affect your scale weight loss. (See "Muscle Weighs More Than Fat..." and "Water-Weight Fluctuation" on pages 21–23.)

What You Will See and Feel

After three weeks of working out, even at fifty or more pounds overweight, you will begin to see some definition in your upper back and shoulder area, but it will be very slight because fat obscures this area when you are extremely overweight. You may also be able to see a slight curve in biceps muscle, and it will feel harder.

If you are on the higher end of the scale, you may not see anything at all in three weeks, but you'll sense that you are tighter. When you touch your body, it will still feel soft because the fat is covering the developing muscles. But your mind will sense that there is strength and firmness forming under the fat.

In six weeks definition will continue in your shoulders and upper back.

Your biceps muscle will begin to appear, and they will feel a lot firmer to the touch. You will be able to make a muscle, and people will begin to be impressed. Your body may begin to feel slightly harder to the touch, depending upon how overweight you are. Your triceps will begin to show some change as the fat diminishes and muscle begins to form. Your stomach and buttocks will begin to go down in size, and your thighs will begin to feel firmer.

In three months definition will continue in your upper back and shoulder area, and your biceps will continue to tighten and be more impressive. Your triceps will show significant change and will not jiggle nearly as much. They may not jiggle at all, depending upon how much more fat is covering the developing muscles. Your stomach will be significantly reduced. Your buttocks will be higher and smaller, and you may begin to see a muscle developing in your front thigh.

In six months, if you were only fifty pounds overweight, you may be nearly at your goal. If you were closer to a hundred pounds overweight, it will take you another six months or slightly longer to reach your goal. But under the fluffy fat, firm, sensual muscles will continue to form, so that in a year or slightly longer, when all of the fat is gone, your tight, toned, well-defined body will be revealed.

If you are very much overweight, the rule of thumb is this: the more overweight you are, the more fat you have covering the muscles and the longer it will take to see the muscles that are forming under the fat. Be patient. Keep working. Have faith. It works as surely as the law of gravity. It's a science. There are no exceptions to the rule. If you follow the low-fat eating plan and work with the weights as described in this program, you will lose your fat and become firm and have feminine muscularity. It cannot fail any more than the law of gravity can cease to work. Believe it. It's true.

Don't Be Afraid That Muscles Under the Fat Will Make You Look "Fatter"

The kind of muscles that you will be forming with this workout are small, sensual muscles that take up a lot less space than the fat you will be losing. You will by no means look bigger just because you are working out. In fact, you will look smaller because your body will begin to be condensed.

So if you are very much overweight, please don't think for a moment that you should wait until you have lost the weight before you start working out. That would be a big mistake. The idea is to put firm, shapely muscles under the fat so that as your fat begins to melt away, your muscles will begin to show, and when all of the fat is gone, your firm, shapely body will be there—and not a sagging "skinny-fat" body!

WHAT IF YOU ARE NOT OVERWEIGHT BUT ARE A "SKINNY FAT"

Perhaps you are one of those ladies who looks great in clothing—who is not overweight but who is just "out of shape." What can you expect from this workout, and do you have to follow the diet in chapter 9?

Lucky you. You can continue to eat what you have been eating—unless of course you realize that your diet is not nutritious and wish to alter it for health reasons.

All you have to do is follow the workout. You can expect to see the same pattern of results as described under the section entitled "What You Will See and Feel" for those who are one to ten pounds overweight. Your weight may go up a pound or two after a few weeks of working out because you will be replacing fat with muscle (read "Muscle Weighs More Than Fat..." on page 21), but you will look tighter, feel firmer, and be more defined. You must get over your obsession with the scale, because now your entire body composition will change.

HEIGHT-WEIGHT CHARTS

As you might have guessed by now, I am not a believer in height-weight charts, but I know we are so conditioned to monitoring and measuring ourselves that I am going to indulge you and provide you with such a guideline. There are, however, a few things you must know in order to find your "ideal" weight on the chart.

The first thing that must be considered when measuring yourself against a height-weight chart is your bone structure, which is a combination of your frame and your height—in other words, your skeleton. Your bone structure determines the basic silhouette of your body without excess fat. Your frame refers to the size of your bones and the way they are placed, irrespective of your height.

We are basically stuck with our bone structure. In fact, we can do nothing to increase or reduce the size of our bones or the way they are placed, but we can do something about what we put on those bones. We can reduce the fat and increase the muscle and affect the shape and definition of those muscles so as to make ourselves appear a lot more shapely and aesthetically pleasing than we would be otherwise. In fact, this has been the area of expertise of bodybuilders—the experts from whom I learn most of my secrets!

If you are tall, you are luckier than shorter women, because your weight is spread over a larger area. A shorter-framed woman must keep her weight lower than you, because after a point she has nowhere to go with the weight but out—while you, a taller-framed woman, can hide the weight over a greater area. As I've mentioned so many times before, on television shows and in my books, were it not for this workout, I would look like so many members of my genetically short family of Russian descent: like a box on wheels.

A Sample Height-Weight Chart

The following height-weight chart is a guideline for those of you who are curious or who feel more comfortable monitoring yourself by weight. I never look at such charts, but I will indulge you if you must.

Before you look at the chart, determine your frame. Then you will be able to see whether or not you are within the range of weight suggested for your height. You will need a partner to help you determine your frame.

FRAME DETERMINATION CHART

Height	Space Between Elbow Bones
4'11"–5'5"	2¼"–2½"
5'6"–5'11"	2⅜"–2⅝"
6'0" and taller	2½"–2¾"

Extend your arm and bend your forearm upward at a 90-degree angle. Turn the inside of your wrist toward your body and extend your fingers straight out. Place the thumb and index fingers of your other hand on the bones that protrude on either side of your elbow. Have your partner take a ruler and measure the space between your fingers. (If you try to do this yourself, by the time you move your fingers away from your elbow area, you will probably have moved your fingers and lost the measurement. It's better, for the sake of accuracy, to use a partner.)

After you have gotten the measurement, compare it to those listed in the above frame determination chart, which gives the frame determination for medium-framed women. If your measurements fall within the range of the chart, you are medium framed. If they fall below those given in the chart, you are a small-framed woman, and if they are higher, you are a large-framed woman.

Now you are ready to find your ideal weight range on the height-weight chart. For your convenience the chart is to be read exactly as it is. No allowance is made for clothing or shoes because I don't want you to have to calculate anything! In other words, I assume you are weighing yourself *in the nude and in bare feet*!

Height-Weight Chart

Height		Small Frame	Medium Frame	Large Frame
Feet	Inches			
4	11	99–108	106–118	115–128
5	0	100–110	108–120	117–131
5	1	101–112	110–123	119–134
5	2	103–115	112–126	122–137
5	3	105–118	115–129	125–140
5	4	108–121	118–132	128–144
5	5	111–124	121–135	131–148
5	6	114–127	124–138	134–153
5	7	117–130	127–141	137–156
5	8	120–133	130–144	140–160
5	9	123–136	133–147	143–166
5	10	126–139	136–150	146–167
5	11	129–142	139–153	159–170
6	0	132–145	142–156	152–173

As you will notice, there is quite a large weight-range allowance. But we will shorten the range. To calculate whether or not you're overweight, find yourself on the chart by first identifying your frame. I'll use myself as an example. I am five feet tall and medium framed. My weight range allows me to fall between a low weight of 108 pounds and a high weight of 120 pounds. How do I know where I belong? It's easy. Before I had muscles, I looked best at the low range of my weight allowance, 108 to 110. In fact, I looked fat if I reached 125 pounds. Now that I have muscles, I would appear to be anorexic at 108 pounds. My ideal lowest weight is now 114–116 pounds, and in the cover and exercise photographs of this book, my weight is 116 pounds! My ideal highest weight is still 120 pounds, but now I can even get away with being as high as 126 pounds and still look good!

Now let's talk about you. Since you do not have significant muscles at this point (I assume), your ideal weight will probably be closer to the lower end of your range. For example, if you are a medium-framed woman of five feet five inches, your ideal weight at this point may be between 121 and 123. But as time goes by, and as you work out and change your body composition to more muscle and less fat, you will be able to weigh more without being overweight. Your ideal weight range will eventually be between 127 and 132, and you will probably even get away with being 137 and still look good. You don't believe me now, but just wait and see! In a year you will look thinner at 127 than you did when you were 121!

WHAT DOES AGE HAVE TO DO WITH IT? GOOD NEWS—NOT MUCH!

In the past I have stated that it may take you a little longer to build muscle if you are over thirty, but I am now delighted to say that research shows no proof whatsoever that it is more difficult to add muscle as you get older. In fact, recent studies show that there is absolutely no difference in the body's ability to put on muscle as you work with weights at any age.

Speed and alacrity are affected by age, but not the ability to build muscle. Strength also decreases with age, but that is due to muscle atrophy. While you can do nothing about loss of some speed and some alacrity, you can do something about muscle atrophy and, in fact, are doing it by working with this program. If you are weak now, in time you will overcome the strength problem and may soon be stronger than women ten years younger than you!

So good news, ladies: you will progress as fast as any younger person when you work out with weights!

By now you may be thinking, "Who is she kidding? We all know that young people seem to literally jump into shape the moment they begin working out." Yes. It does seem that way, and for a very good reason. You see, younger people have naturally better developed muscles (their muscles have not yet begun to atrophy), so when they begin working out and their muscles become even better developed, the overall effect appears to be more dramatic. They have not made more progress than an older person, but the results are more impressive because they had more to begin with.

There is one factor that may cause a younger person to at first actually progress faster than an older person, and that is strength and energy. In the beginning younger people usually have more strength and energy than older people because older people have often neglected their muscles for years, and their muscles have atrophied and have become weaker. If this is the case, younger people will naturally work harder and with more energy in the beginning. It will take an older person a while to replace lost muscle before she has the strength to work as hard as a younger person. But after a few months of using this program, an older person begins to catch up and in time does catch up, and the strength and energy factor may be completely eliminated. Some women are actually stronger and more energetic than women ten to twenty or more years younger than they are. I am one of them!

SPEEDING UP THE PROCESS

The regular Bottoms Up! Workout will get you to your goal in about twelve weeks or twenty-four workout hours (six months or a year if you are extremely overweight or have severely neglected your body; but don't worry—you'll get there). You can go faster or slower if you wish, by adding or subtracting from the program. These plans will be discussed in chapters 6 and 8.

PSYCHOLOGICAL PREPARATION

There are several very important things to do before you start the workout:

1. Read this book from cover to cover.

Underline anything that strikes your fancy. Write comments in margins and question marks near things you don't understand. (You may write to me with questions on anything that is not clear. My address is on page 283. Enclose a stamped, self-addressed envelope and I will personally answer you.)

After reviewing chapter 2 and noting the guidelines of what you can expect based upon the shape you are in now, set a goal date and mark it on the calendar. Setting a goal is a key point, because as I mention time and again in all of my fitness books, the mind is like a homing torpedo: when you give it a specific goal, it will zigzag its way around obstacles to get to that goal. After you've set your goal date, at least once a week, stand in front of the mirror and "tell" your body to get into shape by that target date. If no one is around, say it out loud.

2. Give your body the break it has been begging for.

Make up your mind to maintain it the way you do your teeth, your skin, and your hair. You take time to brush and floss your teeth, to shower, and to shampoo and condition your hair. Realize that just such a small investment of time in your body (twenty to thirty minutes a day) will net you the following:

- **Peace of mind.** You will like the way you look and you will release your psychological energy for creative projects and personal relationships. You will reinvest the energy you used to spend in self-condemnation and apologizing to others for your body, and become more successful in every area of life.

- **Increased self-esteem.** You will like yourself better for having made your outer appearance match more closely your beautiful inner self (your soul).

- **Increased energy.** Your strength will give you more energy, and you'll accomplish more in a given day without feeling tired.

- **Improved health.** Your heart and lungs will be healthier (the aerobic effect and the low-fat diet play a part here).

- **Looking and feeling younger and sexier longer—much longer.** Your bones and muscles will youthe (by working with the weights), and your body will be shapely and sensual. I hate to think of how I would look and feel right now if I didn't work out. I'm pushing fifty, and I look better than I did when I was in my twenties.

3. Realize that it is not too late.

No matter how fat or old you are, you're a perfect candidate for this program. As long as your body hasn't quit on you yet (and it hasn't if you're still breathing), you can improve it with time and self-discipline.

4. Make a six-month commitment to this program.

Although you will see changes in three weeks and dramatic results in three months, I want a six-month commitment from you because it takes that long to establish a lifetime habit. After that you won't want to quit. You will have incorporated the workout into your life the way you do brushing your teeth or taking a shower.

What are you really gambling? Twenty to thirty minutes a day against a lifetime of health and beauty and peace of mind. But it will work. If it doesn't, please write to me immediately because I'm going to put you in "Vedral's Believe It or Not!"

In conclusion, think of it this way: We spend hours keeping our property in shape. We mow our lawns, polish our furniture, tend our gardens, have our cars tuned up, ensure that our clothing is dry-cleaned and in good repair and that our office equipment is in optimum working order. But when it comes to our physical bodies, the only "property" we own that cannot be replaced, we foolishly neglect them. Are we out of our minds? Sometimes I wonder.

So let's stop making excuses and cruelly neglecting our bodies. All I'm asking for is a twenty- to thirty-minute daily commitment, and if you don't have that much time, I'll settle for four twenty-minute weekly sessions (this is discussed in chapter 8).

SEVEN WORKOUT SAVERS

Before you begin the workout, I want to give you some tips that will head off trouble before it comes.

1. Answer yourself back.

After you read this book and become excited about the workout and resolve to "go for it," you may experience some negative thoughts. For example, a little voice in the back of your mind may say to you, "Who are you trying to fool? Look how many times you tried to get in shape and failed. What makes you think you can succeed this time?"

When such thoughts assail you, don't just sit there and take it. Learn to answer yourself back. For example, to the above negative thought, you might say, "So what if I failed before. The road to success is often paved with failure." To further back yourself up, you might think of Woody Allen, who failed motion picture production at NYU and CCNY and yet became more than a little successful in the movie business! You can even think of Thomas Edison, who failed hundreds of times before he eventually found the combination that led him to the invention of the incandescent light bulb. Or you can think of me. I failed at hundreds of shape-up programs until, in my forties, I discovered the weight training methods described in this book.

No matter what the negative thought—whether it be "But you're too old" or "You're too lazy" or "Why waste your time"—don't just bend your back and take the blows. Instead, answer yourself back, and defy the negative voice until it retreats.

2. Make a plan A and a plan B.

One of the more important things—if not *the* most important thing—you can do for yourself if you want your workout to succeed is to set a regular workout time for yourself (a plan A) and an alternate workout time (a plan B) to be used when the regular time is inconvenient.

You will use plan A most of the time, but in case something comes up, you will go into plan B until plan A again becomes feasible.

Your plan A may be to work out in the morning. This is ideal because if you get it done at that time, it's over with and you don't have to think about it again until the next day. Also, in the morning, right after you wake up, you don't have time to analyze the situation to death. You just hop out of bed, wash your face and brush your teeth, take a drink of water, and pick up the dumbbells. Before you know it, you're working out, and twenty to thirty minutes later it's over. You don't even know what happened until later, on the way to work, you realize, "Wow. I already worked out." Amazingly, you also have more energy for the day when you work out in the morning.

Unfortunately, many of us don't have the luxury of being able to work out in the morning. Perhaps we're already required to get up at the crack of dawn in order to be at work early or to tend to small children. In such cases we will have to find the next best time. Analyze your week and find a spot of time when you are free every day. Perhaps it will be lunchtime for you, and you can work out in a spare room in your office. (All you need are three sets of dumbbells and a bench. You can bring them in yourself if your boss won't spring for them.)

You may have to do what I had to do for a couple of years: work out the minute you get home from a long, hard day at work. I would walk in the door, take off my clothing and put on an old pair of shorts and a T-shirt, pick up the dumbbells, and start. Twenty minutes later it was over. Then I checked my answering machine, started dinner, and perhaps turned on the TV.

You may have to work out just before bed, when everyone is tucked in and you have time to yourself. Not the ideal time—but better, much better, than nothing if it's your only free time. (So your metabolism will be up for an hour or two into your sleep and you'll sleep lightly, but you'll be burning fat while you do that, and you'll love yourself for not letting anything get in your way.)

What about plan B? Plan B is your second choice. For example, using the above illustration, the ideal plan is doing it first thing in the morning. Suppose your life-style allows that because you get up at 7:00 A.M. for work and are willing to get up at 6:30 in order to work out. But suppose one day you have to go to the office earlier than usual and are not willing to get up at 6:00. Then think ahead with a plan B and follow it. Again, using the above example, you may have to work out the minute you get home from work. This is your plan B. You've already figured it out—if plan A fails, you will switch gears and go into plan B for that day. You don't resent it but instead are delighted that you feel in control. You realize that you have the power over your life. Circumstances cannot stop you. You're the boss.

So make up a schedule with plans A and B. See chapter 8 for further details on planning your workout.

3. Be flexible.

When it comes to flexibility, I've had to learn some hard lessons, because I tend to be very rigid. I hate it when anything dares to intrude on my routine or my plans. But life has a way of throwing curves our way, so I've had to learn how to be flexible. Sometimes my plans A and B are no longer feasible, and I have to invent creative ways to find time to work out—new plans A and B that might themselves be interrupted.

It may happen to you. If your life is suddenly turned upside down, you can still find a way to work out. Suppose for example that an elderly parent has moved into your home and you have now lost your workout space. You have no basement. Every corner of your home is occupied. If need be, put the bench in your living room and the weights under your couch. The living room, in fact, is an ideal place for your workout equipment, because working out will increase the quality of your life and may even extend it! Which is more important: a picture-book living room or a functioning living room that can house the vital equipment that will greatly enhance your life?

I could go on and on and tell of all the "impossible" situations that people I've heard from—readers of my fitness books—have had to overcome in order to pursue their workout. I think of these obstacles as a test of will and determination, because in the end the people who have figured out ways to get around the obstacles and have continued to work out in spite of the odds are those who have made the most progress.

4. Pick yourself up and start all over again.

One of the most common reasons for quitting a workout is the failure to work out for a few days or even for a week or two. Suppose you were well on your way to a routine, having worked out for three weeks; then suddenly you get the flu and are in bed for a week. When you recover, you feel discouraged, because now you haven't worked out for a week. You say to yourself, "Forget it. You just can't do it." Stop the music right there. Instead of saying "Forget it," say "OK. I'll have to pick myself up, brush myself off, and start all over again." Then set a new "start date" and give it another go.

I don't care if you start and stop ten times in a year, as long as you start again. Even if you made a hundred false starts, it wouldn't matter. As long as you start again, sooner or later you'll catch on and stick with it. One day, just the way you suddenly found yourself riding the two-wheeler after a hundred falls, you'll be working out without thinking about it. It will be as natural to you as something you've done all of your life. But you have to give it time.

5. Sublimate frustration, depression, and anger into the workout.

There will be days when you're just not in the mood to work out. Perhaps you've had a hard day at work and your children are driving you crazy. The roof is leaking, and you don't know where you're going to get the money to pay for the repair. With all of this, you stub your toe and it really hurts. You feel like sitting in front of the TV and eating all evening instead of working out. Instead of letting that frustration cause you to fail in your workout, use it to drive you through it. Say to yourself, "I couldn't control the leak in the roof or the way my boss spoke to me, but I can

39

control whether or not I work out." Then pick up the weights and just do it. After you have finished, you will feel better about your life—you will feel more in control.

If you are depressed and just don't have the energy to move, much less work out, you will have to pick up the dumbbells by an act of will and begin to move them from point A to point B. In five minutes you'll start to feel a little better, and in ten minutes you'll feel a lot better. By the time you finish, you'll wonder where the depression went. Endorphines (natural opiates) produced by the body will have reached your brain during the workout and will have lifted your spirits the same way a drug or a drink would do—only without the negative aftereffects.

If you are angry, instead of kicking the wall or telling someone off, work out. At least after you have finished, you will have accomplished something positive instead of having done damage.

Anger is energy and just like electricity it can be used to destroy or to create. Electricity can electrocute you or it can run a power plant. Sublimate your anger—channel it into the workout and see positive results for your efforts. And there's a bonus in this, too. By the time you finish working out, your anger will be greatly reduced because you will have taken out your frustration on the weights!

6. Visualize—in the mirror, while working out, and to head off trouble.

Help yourself get to your goal by picturing yourself the way you want to look. Stand in front of the mirror in the nude and imagine your body evolving into the shape you have in mind. To help yourself in this effort, take a photograph of yourself and draw over it with magic marker, reshaping your body into its near-perfect form. Make your thighs the size you want them, shape your shoulders and arms the way you dream that they should look. Flatten your stomach and put the lines of definition where they should go. Take a rear-view photo, too, and mark that into shape. Every day look in the mirror and tell your body to get into its ideal shape.

Don't forget to visualize while you are working out. From time to time, as you are performing the repetitions of a specific exercise, picture that body part being reshaped. See the fat melting away as you move the weight, and imagine a firm, sensual muscle being formed. Tell your working body part to get tight and toned.

In order to head off trouble both in the workout and the eating department, do some "advance" visualization. Picture yourself getting up in the morning and being tempted not to work out. Then picture yourself remembering how bad you will feel later in the day when you realize that you didn't work out, and imagine yourself going on automatic and doing the workout in spite of yourself. You will find, to your amazement, that this works. The next time you're tempted not to work out, you'll find that you do it anyway. Preconditioning in visualization helps a lot.

Do the same thing when it comes to heading off diet trouble. Picture yourself being tempted to eat a fatty food, and then picture yourself remembering how angry you are when you give in to temptation. Imagine yourself saying, "No. It's not worth it." The next time you are tempted to break your diet, you may find to your surprise that you decide not to do it.

7. Don't let sticking points get you down.

When you first start working out, you may see a lot of progress in the first month, but then, suddenly, everything may seem to stop: the scale may show little change—and may even go up a pound (water retention)—and you may feel as fat and as sluggish as ever. When this happens, no matter what, *keep going*. The body is its own strange machine, and at times it takes a seeming break from progress—but that break is only outward. Inside, changes are being made, only they are not visible at the moment.

It's the same way with the growth of children. Sometimes they seem to be at a standstill, then suddenly they seem to shoot up overnight. Did they really grow three inches overnight? Of course not. So in the same way children grow when no one is monitoring them, you too will make progress if you keep going—when you're not monitoring yourself and when you least expect it.

Whether your sticking point occurs in the beginning of your workout—and you don't see much of a result in the first three weeks—or whether it occurs after a month or two, remember that no matter what, KEEP GOING. In time you will get past the sticking point, and progress will be evident. Time and again women have written to tell me of just such occurrences. They were discouraged and were about to quit when suddenly they began to see results. How thankful they are that they heeded my advice to keep going no matter what.

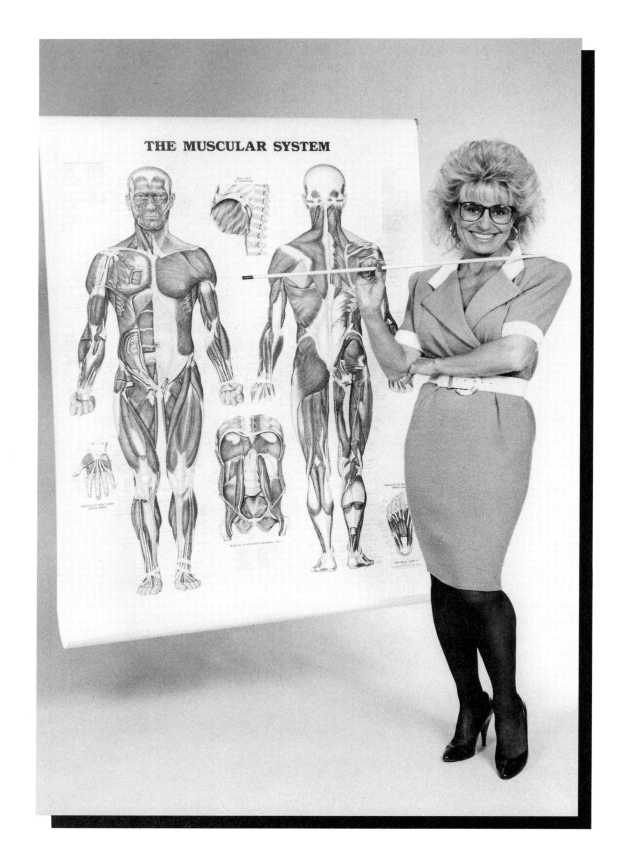

THE MUSCULAR SYSTEM

3

WORKOUT ESSENTIALS

In every fitness program there are certain essentials that one should know in order to have complete insight into what is being accomplished by the program. It is not only important to understand the basic terms that will be repeated again and again in this book, such as *set* and *repetition,* but it is also important to gain a rudimentary understanding of muscles: where they are located, how they function, and how they grow and change as a result of working with weights. It is also important to know a little bit about weight-training techniques, weights, and weight-training equipment in general. These and other related topics will be discussed in this chapter.

You may already be quite familiar with some of the terms mentioned here, but even so, I urge you to give the chapter a quick read-through, because even the terms that are familiar to you will be demonstrated by specific examples from the Bottoms Up! Workout. This chapter, in conjunction with chapters 4 through 6, will help you to understand the workout to the point where you will be able to do it with ease.

TERMS USED IN THE EXERCISE INSTRUCTIONS

As you read the exercise instructions, time and again you will encounter certain expressions. Here is an explanation of the most commonly used terms. You should become quite familiar with them before you start the workout.

An **exercise** is a given movement for a specific muscle, designed to cause that muscle to grow and become stronger. For example, the plié squat is an exercise designed to tighten and tone the inner thigh area.

A **repetition**, or rep, is one complete movement of an exercise, from start, to midpoint, to finish. For example, one repetition of the plié squat involves squatting down from the standing start position (now you are at midpoint) and raising yourself back up to standing (start position). (See page 85 for photographs illustrating this exercise.)

A **set** is a specified number of repetitions of a specific exercise that are performed without a rest. In this workout you will perform fifteen repetitions for each set of your thigh exercises.

An *interset*, or a *twin set*, is a combined set of two exercises of complementary body parts. For example, in this workout you will be doing intersets of thigh and hip/buttock exercises. Specifically, your first interset for your thigh–hip/buttock workout will consist of fifteen repetitions of the plié squat and fifteen repetitions of the standing back leg extension—without a rest between the two exercises. In short, an interset is more than a twin—it is a "Siamese twin." It cannot be split apart.

A **rest** is a pause between sets or exercises. The purpose of the rest is to allow the working muscle enough time to recuperate so that it can efficiently perform the work of the next set. You will be exercising two different body parts in nonstop intersets because a natural rest is provided for the nonworking body part while you are exercising another body part. Yet again, you do need a rest every so often, so an optional zero- to fifteen-second rest is allowed after each interset. (You will be using relatively light weights, so longer rests will not be necessary.)

A **routine** is the specific combination of exercises prescribed for a given body part. In this workout, however, a routine involves the combination of exercises for two given body parts because two are always exercised together. For example, in this workout your chest-shoulder routine consists of twin sets of chest and shoulder exercises: the flat dumbbell press and the seated side lateral; the incline dumbbell fly and the seated alternate dumbbell press; and the cross-bench pullover and the standing alternate front lateral raise.

A **workout** includes all of the exercises to be performed by the exerciser on a given day. For example, in this workout you exercise your lower body on the first workout day: thighs and hips/buttocks, and lower and upper abdominals. Your workout for the second day will include chest and shoulders, biceps and triceps, and back and calves.

The term *workout* can also be used to describe the overall exercise program. For example, the total program in this book is called the Bottoms Up! Workout.

The expression **weight** refers to the *resistance*, or the heaviness, of the weight used in a given exercise. Since this is first and foremost a toning and defining workout—and not a bulk-building program—you will be using lighter weights, or less resistance, than you would in a regular bodybuilding workout. For example, if you are a beginner, you will be using weights varying between one and ten pounds for the entire workout.

Less resistance allows you to work faster and, in turn, to burn more fat and achieve greater definition.

In nearly every exercise instruction you will be told to **flex** your muscle. This means to *contract* the muscle, so that the muscle fibers are shortened as the muscle is squeezed together, and to go a step beyond that by willfully squeezing your working muscle as hard as possible. For example, you will be asked to flex your biceps as you curl your arm upward for your seated simultaneous curl.

You will also notice that quite often, the exercise instructions ask you to feel the **stretch** in your working muscle. Stretching is the opposite of flexing. When a muscle stretches, the muscle fibers lengthen rather than shorten. Using the above example, when performing the seated simultaneous biceps curl, you will be asked to feel the stretch in your biceps as you uncurl your arms and extend them straight down.

TECHNIQUES USED IN THIS WORKOUT

In addition to the specific expressions that you will encounter in the exercise instructions, there are some expressions of technique that will apply to your overall workout. They are explained in the following paragraphs.

An **aerobic** exercise is a physical fitness activity that causes your pulse to reach 60 to 80 percent of its capacity and to stay there for twenty minutes or longer.

You can determine your maximum pulse rate by subtracting your age from 220. If you perform this workout as prescribed, you will be well within the aerobic range. It isn't necessary to continually test your pulse. This can lead to excessive self-consciousness.

While an aerobic activity is sustained by the body's continual supply of oxygen, an **anaerobic** activity is not. An anaerobic activity is far too demanding to be supported by the body's natural oxygen supply, so an oxygen debt is accrued. When this happens, the exerciser is forced to take a rest in order to literally catch her breath. Power lifting is an example of an anaerobic activity.

Although regular weight training has traditionally also been considered to be an anaerobic activity, it becomes an aerobic activity if it is done as described in this workout. How can this be? The participant is asked to perform a continual, steady flow of movements with the utilization of comparatively light weights, so the body is able to maintain enough oxygen to sustain the activity. Although the Bottoms Up! Workout is, in and of itself, aerobic, you will be asked to do several weekly aerobic sessions of your choice in order to burn additional fat and to strengthen your heart and lungs for the workout itself.

Intensity is the degree of difficulty of the exercise program you are following. Intensity can be increased by increasing the number of repetitions, increasing the load of weight, or reducing the rest periods allowed between sets and between exercises. *Bottoms-Up!* prescribes a high-intensity program because you are allowed only a few short, optional rests and because you are performing a relatively high number of repetitions. (You will be exercising two different body parts simultaneously, often doing thirty repetitions before you are allowed to rest—fifteen repetitions for each of two body parts.)

Muscle isolation is the method of exercising a body part completely and independently of other body parts. In order to ensure maximum shaping and strengthening of a given body part, it is necessary to provide that body part with uninterrupted work. In the past I have said that it is not OK to do one exercise for a given body part, and then to switch to an exercise for another body part. Now I am telling you to do just that. Is there a contradiction here? Not at all. You must never switch around at random and perform exercises for, say, shoulders, then back, then thighs, then triceps, and so on. Too much time would lapse between exercises for a given body part, and that body part would not receive enough of a challenge to grow and develop.

Bottoms Up! asks you to work within a very tight, carefully planned framework of switching back and forth between two related body parts with virtually no rest. Very little time elapses between sets for a given body part (in fact, less time than elapses during a regular bodybuilding workout, which requires one to rest at least forty-five seconds between sets). The end result is muscle isolation plus!

The **split routine** is the working of a given number of body parts on workout day one, and a given number of other body parts on workout day two, and so on. A routine can be split into two or three workout days. *Bottoms Up!* follows the two-day split.

The purpose of the split routine is to allow the exercised muscle the required forty-eight hours rest before it is challenged again. The community of athletic experts generally agrees that most muscles need forty-eight hours to recuperate from a workout. (Abdominal muscles are an exception to this rule.) If not allowed this amount of rest time, a muscle may become exhausted from overtraining, and development may be hindered or reversed.

The split routine allows you to work out every day if you so choose because you never exercise the same body parts on two consecutive days. In this workout the routine is split into the lower and middle body workout on workout day one, and the upper body workout on workout day two.

A **regular pyramid system** of weight training involves the adding of weight to each set with a simultaneous reduction of repetitions until a peak is achieved, and then the reduction of weight on each set with a simultaneous addition of reps until the starting amount of weight and reps is reached. The system is more readily understood with a simple example.

Set 1: twelve repetitions, three pounds
Set 2: ten repetitions, five pounds
Set 3: eight repetitions, eight pounds
Set 4: ten repetitions, five pounds
Set 5: twelve repetitions, three pounds

Fitness experts and bodybuilders use the regular pyramid system as a method of shocking the muscles into working harder. For our purposes the **modified pyramid system** is superior to the regular pyramid system, because it does not allow the muscle to become exhausted. The modified pyramid system asks you to work up to the peak of the pyramid and stop there. In other words, you add weight to each set and simultaneously reduce the repetitions for each set until you reach the peak of the pyramid, but you do not descend the pyramid. Here is an example of the modified pyramid system for the chest-shoulder routine.

Set 1: twelve repetitions, three pounds
Set 2: ten repetitions, five pounds
Set 3: eight repetitions, eight pounds

(As will be explained later, the specific weights you use will depend upon your present level of fitness.)

Progression refers to the occasional adding of weight to specific exercises when the weight being used for those exercises is no longer enough of a challenge. For example, after a while (perhaps a month) it will seem to you that the weights you are using in a routine in this workout are too easy to lift. When this happens, in order to make progress and continue to see your muscles develop, you must add weight to those exercises. For example, if your biceps-triceps routine seems to be too easy, you will switch to five, eight, and ten pounds.

HOW MUSCLES AND BONES GROW

When a muscle contracts against resistance with sufficient force, the muscle cells cope with that strain by synthesizing protein. When this happens, the muscle cells enlarge and grow stronger. (Tendons and ligaments, tissue that connects muscle and bone are also made stronger when challenged by significant resistance.)

Bone is living tissue composed of calcium phosphate and the protein collagen. Within the bone lie hundreds of concentric rings called haversian canals. When significant force is exerted upon a bone to which a working muscle is attached, an increased blood flow is sent surging through the bone, and eventually, the bone thickens as the blood carries nutrients to the bone-building cells. In addition, the stress upon the bone caused by lifting weights causes an electrical charge to shoot through the haversian canals and to further stimulate the cells of the bone. The combination of increased blood flow and the stimulating electrical charge is what causes bones to thicken.

Most women lose up to 10 percent of their bone mass by the time they are fifty, and another 10 percent by the time they are seventy. Men lose about half that amount. As has been discussed in chapter 1, weight training can reverse bone loss. For example, I have not lost any bone, and I am nearly fifty! In fact, I now have thicker bones than I had when I was thirty!

EXPRESSIONS DESCRIBING THE WAY YOUR MUSCLES WILL GROW

As you continue to work out, your body will begin to evolve into its perfect form. You will begin to see muscle growth and muscle mass as your muscularity increases. You will add definition to your muscles, and they may even at times appear "ripped." As your body fat continues to decrease, your muscle density will increase. What does all of this mean in terms of the Bottoms Up! Workout?

Muscle mass is the actual size of a given muscle. As you continue to use the Bottoms Up! Workout, you will experience **muscle growth** (hypertrophy). This takes place over a period of time when the muscle is forced to work harder than usual on a regular basis. In order to grow extremely large, a muscle must be required to lift very heavy weights over a period of time, but in order to grow at all and to have even feminine muscularity, the muscles must be regularly challenged with moderate weights over a period of time.

Muscularity, as opposed to muscle mass, depicts the quantity of muscle as opposed to fat. As you continue to do the Bottoms Up! Workout and to follow the low-fat eating plan, your muscularity will increase. In other words, your body will evolve into being composed of more muscle and less fat than was previously the case.

While all of this is happening, you will begin to see **definition** in your muscles. Definition is recognized by clearly delineated lines. For example, after working out for about three months, you will notice pretty lines of definition in your shoulders and upper back area.

A **"ripped"** muscle is a muscle that has extreme definition and has taken on a look of striation. An example of ripped muscles can be seen on a bodybuilder who has slender lines separating his abdominal muscles. In general, these lines make the muscle more attractive in appearance and can even help to draw attention away from body faults. (For example, the definition you will achieve in your side abdominal area by doing the oblique crunch will put lines of definition along your side abdominals and help to make your waist appear smaller.)

A muscle is said to have **density** when it is hard. In order to achieve density, or hardness, it is necessary to work intensely, as described in this workout, and in addition, to eliminate excess body fat.

Symmetry is a term depicting the aesthetic balance and proportion of muscles in relationship to other muscles on the body. This workout is designed to help create near-perfect symmetry for your body. (There is no such thing as perfect symmetry on the human body. Our profile is proof of this. Most of us take a better photograph on one side of the face than on the other.)

If you decide to exercise only one body part to the exclusion of all others, you will move further away from body symmetry. If the cartoon character Popeye were not fictitious, I would ask him to stop doing arm exercises and to start working his chest, shoulder, and back muscles!

EQUIPMENT AND OPTIONAL EQUIPMENT USED IN THIS WORKOUT

Your equipment for this workout will be limited to dumbbells and a bench. (You can perform the bench exercises at the edge of a chair, bed, or sofa if you cannot purchase a bench, but a bench is safer and better.) Those of you who opt to do the barbell exercises will need a barbell and some plates. Those of you who opt to do the gym workout will want to know the advantages and disadvantage of free weights as compared to machines.

The **flat exercise bench** is a structure built specifically for the purpose of exercise. It is a long, narrow, padded bench that is parallel to the floor.

The **incline exercise bench** is the same as a flat bench, only it can be raised to an incline (as high as a 45-degree angle). Since you will need both flat and incline exercise benches for this workout, it's a good idea to purchase a flat bench that can be raised to an incline. Another possibility is to buy a flat bench and put two taped-together telephone directories under the foot of the bench when you do incline exercises.

Free weights are handheld weights that can be carried about. Free weights include dumbbells, barbells, and exercise plates.

A **dumbbell** is a short bar (usually made of metal) that can be held in one hand and that has a raised section on either end. Most dumbbells have a permanently fixed weight on either end. (I do not recommend the kind with removable plates. It takes too long to take them apart for readjustment, and they often loosen while you are using them.)

A **barbell** is a metal bar that is held in both hands and that holds various weights on either end. Barbells come in weights from fifteen to forty-five pounds. You will need a barbell and a few very light plates for this workout, but only if you choose to do the exercise variations.

Plates are disk-shaped weights that can be placed on either end of the barbell. They come in sizes as light as one and a quarter pounds and go as high as forty-five pounds. If you choose to use the alternative barbell exercises, I suggest that you purchase a 15- to 25-pound barbell and sets of two-and-a-half–pound, five-pound, and ten-pound plates. You probably won't need more than that.

A **collar** is the device placed on either end of the barbell after the plates are added. Collars are used to keep the plates from sliding off the barbell. Placing and removing collars is time-consuming. If you're anything like I am, you will learn to balance the barbell so that the weights do not fall off. However, for 100 percent safety, use the collars.

The **exercise machine** is designed to challenge one or more specific body parts. Years ago, the Nautilus machine and the Universal machine were virtually the only available machines. Today, there are hundreds of brand-name machines, such as Cybex, Marcy, Paramount, etc.

WHY FREE WEIGHTS ARE SUPERIOR TO MACHINES FOR THE PURPOSE OF THIS WORKOUT

In general there are distinct advantages in using free weights as opposed to using machines—and several specific advantages for the purpose of this workout.

First, you can achieve greater flexibility by using free weights than you can by using machines. You can fit the weights to your size, but not the machines, no matter how diligently you adjust them. The fact is, most machines are not made to accommodate smaller people, and this boils down to *women*, because in general, compared to men, women are small people!

You can effect muscle change more efficiently with free weights since, with them, you are in complete control of the weight and can monitor the velocity and resistance of each repetition. Machines do not allow for full natural movements, no matter how efficient they are. The fact is, machines do just a little bit of the work for you, and that, in my opinion, is why so many people love to use them.

Free weights are more convenient than machines. Whether you're working out in a gym or at home, they can be carried to a corner and hoarded until one's workout is complete.

Finally, and perhaps most important, free weights are more versatile. For example, you can work all nine body parts by using a mere set of dumbbells. In order to work all nine body parts using machines, you would need at least twelve machines to complete your workout. (Remember, you must do at least three exercises per body part to get a complete workout. That means at least twenty-seven different exercises. Most exercise machines provide two or three exercises; some provide more.)

The advantages that machines have over free weights do not apply to this workout. For example, machines are usually considered to be safer than free weights for lifting heavy weights because the machine's weights are controlled by slides or cams and held in place by retaining pins. If you should drop a heavy weight, the machine would catch it. However, since you will be using very light weights with this workout, you are not likely to drop your weights.

Machines are also said to be more efficient in isolating a muscle group for heavy overload. In other words, a bench press machine can hold 200 pounds of weight, whereas it would be quite awkward to pick up two 100-pound dumbbells. You will not be overloading your muscles in this workout. Free weights are perfect for muscle isolation if you are working with relatively light weights.

There are a few machines that seem to be irreplaceable when it comes to certain body parts. They are the lat pulldown machine and the pulley row machine for the back; and the leg press, the leg extension, and the leg curl machines for the thighs. True, these machines can be eliminated (as they are in this workout) by free weight substitutes, but the machines are preferable if they are available because they allow you to position yourself in a way that you simply cannot achieve with free weights. For this reason, whenever I am in a gym (which is often not for months at a time), I will use them.

WHY YOUR MUSCLES WILL BECOME SORE AS A RESULT OF THIS WORKOUT

Muscle soreness is the result of microscopic tears in the fibers of the ligaments and tendons connecting the muscles, and of the slight internal swelling that accompanies those tears. Experts agree that the tears usually occur during the stretch part of the exercise rather than the flex part—while the muscle fibers are lengthening, yet at the same time trying to contract in order to deal with the work being required of them.

Tears are perfectly normal; they are, in fact, necessary if you're going to make any progress in changing the shape of your body. In fact, if you don't experience any soreness, write to me immediately. I will be concerned!

WHY YOU MUST WORK THROUGH THE SORENESS—NO MATTER WHAT!

Depending upon how gently you break in, you can expect a medium to great amount of soreness the first week and a gradual lessening of soreness over the next three weeks until it is all gone.

If you are sore, the very worst thing you could possibly do would be to stop working out and wait for the soreness to go away. When it comes to muscle soreness, I must woefully deliver the bad news: you must bite the bullet and work through the soreness. The workout itself will serve as a massage for the sore muscles. It helps to relax them as it stretches and flexes them, and encourages the blood to circulate around them.

If you are really "drop dead" sore, you can use lighter weights for a workout or two and then gradually go up to your original weight (in about a week). If you're really "in traction" sore, OK, I'll indulge you. You can do the workout with no weights for a day or two, then use very light weights, and then go back to your regular weights. But under no circumstances are you allowed to take a week off to recuperate. If you do this, you will be back to square one and will experience the same soreness the next time you work out, and will again stop, and so on, until you eventually quit working out.

THE DIFFERENCE BETWEEN INJURY AND SORENESS

When you experience an injury, you know it immediately. Rather than a slow, gradual ache, you feel an immediate, sharp pain that renders you nearly incapable of continuing to work out. The most common injuries in weight training are fascia injuries (tears to the covering of the muscle), stretching and tearing of ligaments, and tendinitis (painful inflammation of a tendon.)

There is little chance of injury with the Bottoms Up! Workout because you will be using light weights—unless of course you ignore the exercise instructions and begin swinging the weights around wildly, pulling and jerking them in an abrupt manner, or using extremely heavy weights.

54

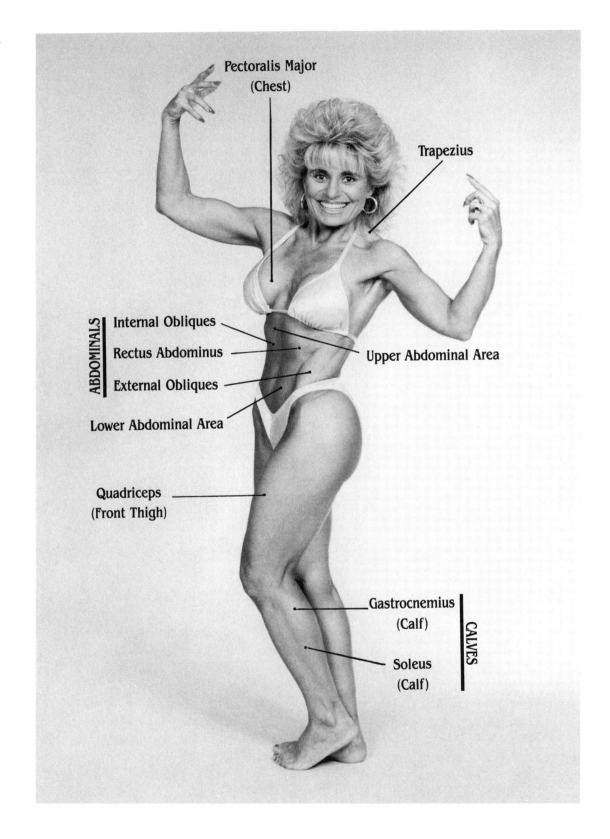

Pectoralis Major
(Chest)

Trapezius

ABDOMINALS

Internal Obliques

Rectus Abdominus

External Obliques

Lower Abdominal Area

Upper Abdominal Area

Quadriceps
(Front Thigh)

Gastrocnemius
(Calf)

CALVES

Soleus
(Calf)

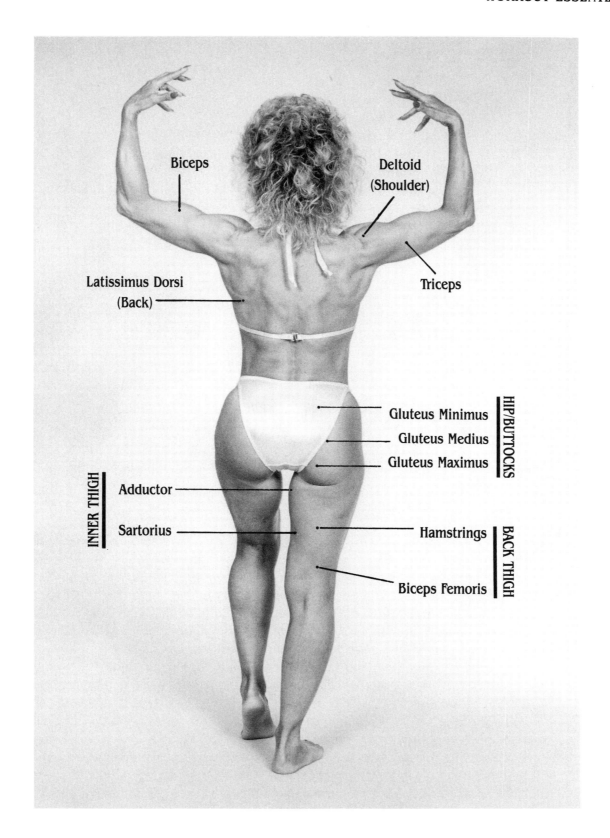

Biceps

Deltoid
(Shoulder)

Latissimus Dorsi
(Back)

Triceps

HIP/BUTTOCKS

Gluteus Minimus

Gluteus Medius

Gluteus Maximus

INNER THIGH

Adductor

Sartorius

Hamstrings

BACK THIGH

Biceps Femoris

DESCRIPTION OF THE MUSCLES INVOLVED IN THIS WORKOUT

In order to visualize properly, you have to know what you are visualizing. For example, when you are exercising your thigh muscles, it would be most helpful to you if you could actually see in your mind the quadriceps (front thigh muscle) developing, and the adductor (inner thigh muscle) becoming firm. If you knew what the muscles looked like and where they were located in your body, you could actually see them in your mind as you worked, and you could mentally tell them to become firm and defined.

For your convenience the following muscle descriptions are given in the order in which you will find them in the exercise chapters. For example, on your first exercise day you will work your thighs (quadriceps), hips/buttocks, and abdominals. These muscle groups are discussed first, in that order. On workout day two you will exercise your chest-shoulder, biceps-triceps, and back-calf muscle groups. They are discussed next, in that order.

Front, Inner, and Back Thigh
(Quadriceps, Sartorius, Adductor, and Biceps Femoris, or Hamstrings)

The quadriceps, or front thigh muscle, does the work of extending your leg from the bent position. It is composed of four muscles: the rectus femorus and the vasti (there are three vasti muscles altogether). The rectus femoris originates on a ridge on the front of the hipbone, while the three vasti muscles originate in various parts of the thigh bone. All four muscles terminate in the knee.

The quadriceps muscle is challenged by the plié squat, the Bugs Bunny lunge, the sissy squat, the leg extension, and the hack squat.

The sartorious runs along the inner thigh, from the hipbone to the inside of the knee. It is the longest muscle in the human body. It functions to rotate the thigh.

The adductor muscles are located on the inner thigh as well. This muscle group originates from the lower pelvic area on the pubis bone and rises to the shaft of the thighbone, where it is inserted. In cooperation with other inner thigh muscles, this muscle group works to flex, rotate, and pull the legs together from a wide stance. This muscle group, in conjunction with the sartorius, is developed by the plié squat, the Bugs Bunny lunge, the sissy squat, the lying inner-thigh scissor.

The back thigh is composed of the biceps femoris and semimembranosus and semitendinosus muscles. Together, this muscle group is called the hamstrings.

The biceps femoris is a two-headed muscle that, in cooperation with two others, the semimembranosus and semitendinosus, works to bend the knee. These muscles originate in the bony area of the pelvis and end along the back of the knee joint. The sissy squat, the hack squat, and the leg curl challenge this muscle.

Hips/Buttocks
(Gluteus Maximus, Gluteus Medius, and Gluteus Minimus)

The largest of the gluteus muscles, the gluteus maximus originates from the iliac crest of the thighbone and runs down to the tailbone. It works to extend and rotate the thigh when extreme force is needed, as in climbing the stairs.

The gluteus medius is located just beneath the gluteus maximus. It functions to raise the leg out to the side and to balance the hips as weight is transferred from one foot to the other.

The gluteus minimus originates on the iliac crest of the hipbone and performs the same function as the gluteus medius. The standing back leg extension, the standing butt squeeze, the straight-leg kick-up, the vertical scissor, the feather kick-up, the prone butt lift, and the lying butt lift all work to tone and shape the gluteus muscles.

Abdominals
(Rectus Abdominus, External Obliques, and Internal Obliques)

The rectus abdominus is an elongated, powerful, segmented muscle that works to pull the torso, or upper body, toward the lower body when sitting up from a lying position. The "abs" originate from the fifth, sixth, and seventh ribs and run vertically across the abdominal wall.

Although the rectus abdominus is technically one long muscle, it is usually considered to be plural for two reasons: the segmented nature of the muscle and the division into upper and lower sections for purposes of exercise. (You will note that upper and lower abdominals are exercised in twin pairs in this workout. While one section of the abdominal area is partially resting, the other section is working.) The knee-in and the bent-knee leg raise exercises challenge the lower abdominal area, and the crunch, the bent-knee sit-up, and the reverse crunch challenge the upper abdominal area.

The external oblique muscles originate at the side of the lower ribs and run diagonally to the rectus abdominus. They are attached to the sheath of fibrous tissue that surrounds the rectus abdominus. These muscles function with other muscles to rotate and flex the torso.

The internal oblique muscles run at right angles to the external obliques and beneath them. It is this angle that forms the shape of the waistline and that determines its size. The greater the slant of the oblique muscles, the narrower the waist.

The oblique crunch challenges the oblique muscles.

Chest
(Pectoralis Major—Pectorals, or "Pecs")

The pectoralis major is a two-headed fan-shaped muscle that lies across the front of the upper chest. The clavicular head, which is the smallest of the two heads, forms the upper pectoral area, while the larger sternal head forms the lower pectoral area. The pectoral muscles originate at the collarbone and run along the breastbone to the cartilage connecting the upper ribs to the breastbone. In women, these muscles are covered by the fatty tissue known as breasts. Breast size can increase only by adding fat to that area, but breast size can appear to increase and to be uplifted if the pectoral muscles are well developed. In addition, well-developed pectoral muscles give the chest muscles definition—in other words, cleavage. The dumbbell press (flat and incline), the dumbbell flye (flat and incline), and the cross-bench pullover all challenge the pectoral muscles.

Shoulder
(Deltoid)

The deltoid is a triangular muscle that resembles an inverted version of the Greek letter delta. It has three parts, which can function independently or as a group: the anterior (front) deltoid, the medial (middle or side) deltoid, and the posterior (rear) deltoid.

The entire deltoid originates in the upper area of the shoulder blade, where it joins the collarbone. The three parts of the muscle weave together and are attached on the bone of the upper arm. One angle drapes over the shoulder area, another points down the arm, weaving around the front of that arm, and the third drapes down the back of the arm.

The anterior deltoid works with the pectoral muscles to lift the arm and to move it forward. The medial deltoid helps to lift the arm sideways, and the posterior deltoid works in conjunction with the latissimus dorsi to extend the arm backward. The seated side lateral, the seated alternate dumbbell press, the standing alternate front lateral raise, the seated bent lateral, and the pee-wee lateral all work to develop and shape the shoulder muscles.

Biceps

The biceps is a two-headed muscle (hence its name) with one short head and one long head. Both heads originate on the cavity of the shoulder blade where the upper-arm bone inserts into the shoulder. The two heads join to form a "hump" about a third of the way down the arm. The other end of the biceps is attached to the bones of the forearm by one connecting tendon.

The biceps works to twist the hand and to flex the arm. The seated simultaneous curl, the standing alternate hammer curl, the seated concentration curl, the seated alternate curl, and the incline simultaneous hammer curl challenge the biceps muscle.

Triceps

The triceps, located on the "other side of the arm" just opposite the biceps, consists of three heads (hence *triceps*). One of the heads attaches to the shoulder blade, while the other two originate from the back side of the upper arm and insert at the elbow.

The longer head of the triceps functions to pull the arm back once it has been moved away from the body, while the other two heads, in conjunction with the longer head, work to extend the arm and the forearm. The close bench triceps press, the flat and incline cross-face triceps extension, the one-arm overhead triceps extension, and the one-arm triceps kickback challenge this muscle.

Back
(Latissimus Dorsi and Trapezius)

The latissimus dorsi originates along the spinal column in the middle of the back and travels upward and sideways to the shoulders, inserting in the front of the upper arm.

The latissimus dorsi help to give the back its V shape, or its width. Well-developed "lats" also help to make a woman's waist appear smaller.

The latissimus dorsi work to pull the shoulder back and downward and the arm toward the body. The leaning one-arm dumbbell row, the seated dumbbell back lateral, and the double-arm reverse row challenge these muscles.

The trapezius is a triangular muscle. It originates along the spine and runs from the back of the neck to the middle of the back. The upper fibers of the trapezius are attached to the collarbone and show up in the neck-shoulder area. For this reason most people think of "traps" as being located only between the neck and shoulder area, when in reality the area that shows here is more like the tip of the iceberg.

The upper trapezius muscles function to shrug the shoulders and pull the head back, while the lower part of the muscle group helps to support the shoulder blade when the arm is raised in an above-the-head position. The upright row and the bent-knee dead lift help to develop this muscle.

Calf
(Gastrocnemius and Soleus)

The gastrocnemius is a two-headed muscle that connects in the middle of the lower leg and ties in with the Achilles tendon. The point where the two muscles are connected, or tied together, form what we see as the calf muscle.

The gastrocnemius helps to bend the knee and flex the foot downward. It works in opposition to the extensor muscles of the lower leg, which pull the foot upward.

The soleus muscle originates on the back of the tibia and head of the fibula bones. It lies just underneath the gastrocnemius muscle but does not pass the knee joint. For this reason, the muscle functions only to flex the foot downward but cannot help to bend the knee. The seated calf raises (angled-in-toe, angled-out-toe, and straight-toe) and standing calf raises (angled-out-toe and straight-toe) all work to challenge this muscle group.

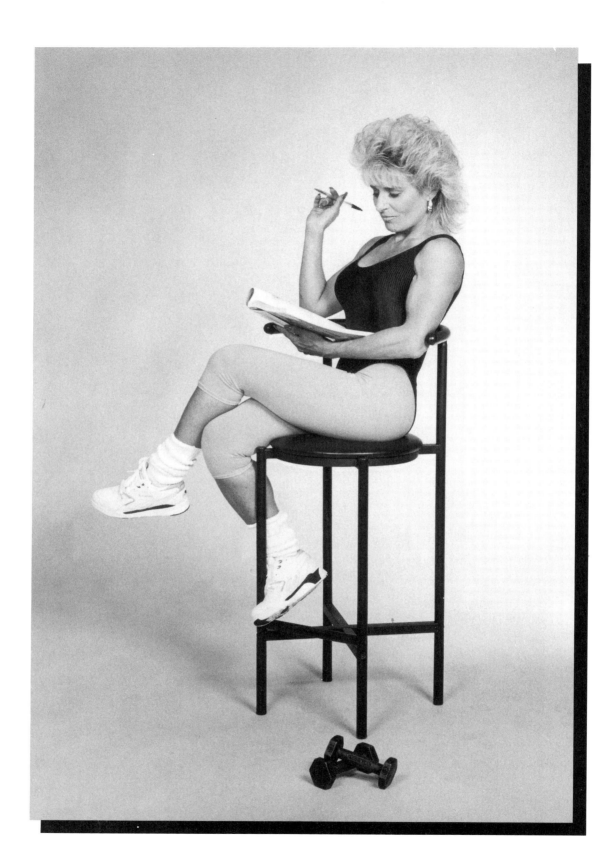

4

HOW TO DO
THE BOTTOMS UP!
WORKOUT

Now that you know what to expect and are familiar with the expressions that will be used over and over again in the workout instructions, it's time to learn how to do the Bottoms Up! Workout. In this chapter you will learn how to perform the intersets that compose this routine, how to use the therapeutic alternatives if you cannot do a specific exercise because of back or knee problems, and how to use the variations if you become bored with a given exercise.

You will also learn how to break in, which depends upon your present condition, and you will be informed about home and gym options.

Sets, repetitions, weights, and other details pertaining to specific workout chapters are discussed in chapters 5 and 6. (For example, you will be doing higher reps for your lower and middle body on workout day one, and you will be doing lower repetitions for your upper body on workout day two.)

How many days a week to work out and various workout plans will be discussed in chapter 8.

THE BALANCE OF THE WORKOUT

You will be doing half of your exercises each workout day. At first, it may not appear that this can be possible, since you are only going to be exercising three body parts on workout day one, and six body parts on workout day two. But when you take a closer look, you can see that on day one you are doing nearly double the exercises for your lower and middle body parts (seven exercises for thighs and hips/buttocks, and five exercises for abdominals), while on day two, you are doing only three exercises for each upper body part. So it evens out. In fact, there are almost exactly the same amount of exercises on each given day: there are nineteen exercises on day one, and eighteen exercises on day two.

The Bottoms Up! Workout—Day One
Lower and Middle Body

On workout day one you will be exercising the following body parts in twin pairs or intersets.

THIGH–HIP BUTTOCK ROUTINE

Thighs	Hips/Buttocks
1. Plié squat (*or* lying one-legged inner-thigh squeeze)	1. Standing back leg extension
2. Bugs Bunny lunge (*or* standing one-legged thigh sweep)	2. Standing butt squeeze
3. Sissy squat (*or* modified sissy squat)	3. Straight-leg kick-up
4. Leg extension	4. Vertical scissor
5. Hack squat (*or* toes-pointed-out leg extension)	5. Feather kick-up
6. Leg curl	6. Prone butt lift
7. Lying inner-thigh scissor	7. Lying butt lift

ABDOMINAL ROUTINE

Lower Abdominals

1. Knee-in (*or* reverse crunch)

2. Bent-knee leg raise (*or* six-inch leg raise)

Upper Abdominals

1. Crunch

2. Bent-knee sit-up (*or* knee-raised crunch)

Side Abdominals (Obliques)

1. Oblique crunch

2. Reverse crunch (*optional*)

The Bottoms Up! Workout—Day Two
Upper Body

On workout day two you will be exercising the following body parts in twin pairs, or intersets.

CHEST-SHOULDER ROUTINE

Chest

1. Flat dumbbell press

2. Incline dumbbell flye

3. Cross-bench pullover

4. Incline dumbbell press (WW)

5. Flat dumbbell flye (T)

Shoulders

1. Seated side lateral

2. Seated alternate dumbbell press

3. Standing alternate front lateral raise

4. Seated bent lateral (WW)

5. Pee-wee lateral (T)

BICEPS-TRICEPS ROUTINE

Biceps

1. Seated simultaneous curl

2. Standing alternate hammer curl

3. Seated concentration curl

4. Seated alternate curl (WW)

5. Incline simultaneous hammer curl (T)

Triceps

1. Close bench triceps press

2. Flat cross-face triceps extension

3. One-arm overhead triceps extension

4. One-arm triceps kickback (WW)

5. Incline cross-face triceps extension (T)

BACK-CALF ROUTINE

Back

1. Leaning one-arm dumbbell row

2. Upright row

3. Seated dumbbell back lateral

4. Double-arm reverse row (WW)

5. Bent-knee dead lift (T)

Calves

1. Seated straight-toe calf raise

2. Standing straight-toe calf raise

3. Seated angled-in-toe calf raise

4. Seated angled-out-toe calf raise (WW)

5. Standing angled-out-toe calf raise (T)

Note: "WW" stands for Wild Woman Workout, and "T" stands for the Terminator Workout. These special workouts will be discussed in chapter 6.

HOW TO DO THE BOTTOMS UP! WORKOUT: WORKING IN INTERSETS

It's easy. You will perform your intersets in the same manner for all twin pairs of exercises—on both workout day one and workout day two. Let me take you through some of the exercises of the thigh–hip buttock routine found in workout day one, and then the exercises for the abdominals routine, also found in day one.

You will do one set of your first thigh exercise, the plié squat, and then without resting you will do one set of the companion hip/buttock exercise, the standing back leg extension. Now you may rest zero to fifteen seconds and do your second set of the plié squat and, without resting, another set of the standing back leg extension. Now you will have completed two full intersets. You may now rest zero to fifteen seconds and then do your final interset of these two exercises. (Remember: There is no rest between the plié squat and the standing back leg extension. These are Siamese twins. They are an interset. They cannot be separated.)

Now you have finished all three sets of your first thigh–hip/buttock exercise combination and are ready to move on to the next thigh–hip/buttock exercise combination. You may rest zero to fifteen seconds and then do your first interset of that exercise combination, the Bugs Bunny lunge and the standing butt squeeze.

Proceeding in the same manner as above, you will do one set of the thigh exercise, the Bugs Bunny lunge, and without resting you will do one set of the hip/buttock exercise, the standing butt squeeze. Then you may rest zero to fifteen seconds and perform your second set of this combination, remembering not to rest until you have completed the interset (both exercises in the combination). Then you may rest zero to fifteen seconds and perform your third and final interset of this combination. Then you may rest zero to fifteen seconds and proceed to your third exercise combination in this exercise group, the sissy squat and the straight-leg kick-up.

You will proceed in this manner, doing both sides of the interset, or twin pair, until you have completed all seven exercises in your thigh–hip/buttock routine.

Now you may take the same zero- to fifteen-second rest and move right along to your abdominal routine. There is no extra rest just because you are starting a new body part. You will be exercising your abdominals in twin pairs of "lower" and "upper" abdominal exercises.

You will do your first set of the lower abdominal exercise, the knee-in, and without resting, the first set of the upper abdominal exercise, the crunch. You may then rest zero to fifteen seconds and do your second interset of this combination. (As always, you will not rest between the two exercises. Remember, intersets are Siamese twins.) You will perform your second interset of that combination and may rest zero to fifteen seconds before going on to complete your third and final interset, the knee-in and the optional reverse crunch.

Now you may rest zero to fifteen seconds and proceed to the next exercise combination, the bent-knee leg raise and the bent-knee sit-up. You will do three intersets for this exercise combination in the same manner as above. Now you will move to the final abdominal exercise, the oblique crunch. This is the only solo exercise in the entire program. You will do three sets of this exercise, resting five to fifteen seconds between sets. (Since you are performing this exercise alone, you will want to rest at least a few seconds to mark the beginning of a new set each time.)

Because this is the only solo exercise, I have offered you the option of pairing it with the reverse crunch. If you choose to do this, you will be doing six exercises for your abdominal area rather than the required five.

You will perform the exercises for your day-two upper-body routine in exactly the same manner as you perform your exercises for day one, working in intersets, or twin pairs, for chest-shoulders, biceps-triceps, and back-calves. Again, these intersets cannot be broken apart, and again, you may take zero- to fifteen-second rests after you perform each interset.

WHAT ABOUT THE RESTS?

You may be wondering about the zero- to fifteen-second rests. Am I telling you that if you don't want to, you don't have to rest at all? That's exactly what I'm saying. You see, this workout is designed to make it possible for you to go nearly nonstop, because the exercises are paired so that you will experience minimum fatigue. Let me explain.

You may be able to speed through your thigh–hip/buttock routine without resting at all, because even though your thighs will be tired after doing an exercise, it won't matter, since you will be doing a hip/buttock exercise right after it, and a hip/buttock exercise provides a nearly complete rest for your thighs. After you complete the hip/buttock half of the interset, you are entitled to a fifteen-second rest, but you may feel as if you've already rested, since your thigh muscles were resting while your hip/buttock muscles were working. You may decide to plunge right ahead and do your second set of the thigh exercise.

How can this be? The fact is, even though you are still working while you exercise your hips/buttocks, your thighs are almost completely resting, so you feel as if you've already had a rest.

What is the advantage of eliminating rests when you feel as if you don't need them? You burn more fat because you are continuing to move. But don't worry. The workout is so intense that even if you take advantage of every single fifteen-second rest, you will still burn vast amounts of fat.

It is most likely that you will have to rest when you do your abdominal and chest-shoulder workouts. Let me explain. When you do a lower abdominal exercise, even though your lower abdominal muscles are doing most of the work, your upper abdominal muscles are doing some of the work and may need a rest before beginning a second interset. The same holds true for chest and shoulder muscles. These muscle groups are closely related in the work that they do. While your chest muscles are working, your shoulder muscles are also working, although not as hard. Most people take full advantage of the optional fifteen-second rests after a chest-shoulder interset.

Biceps and triceps are another matter. Although biceps and triceps are located on either side of the arm, they do different work and are virtually isolated from each other in this respect (see page 59 for how these muscles function). You may be able to breeze through the biceps and triceps workout without resting at all.

Back and calves, the "odd couple" of this program, are a pleasure to exercise, because obviously these muscle groups are completely isolated from each other. When you are working your back, your calves get a complete rest. Therefore, there is no reason why you cannot zoom right through your back-calf routine if you choose to do so—and not rest at all!

BREAKING IN

With all of this talk of breezing and zooming through the workout, it would be easy to forget that it's going to take a little time to break into the workout itself, and a while longer before you'll be able to zip right through it. Exactly how long it will take you to break in will depend upon your exercise conditioning: how much weight training and/or aerobics you have done in the past.

Breaking In If You Have Already Been Working with Weights and Are in Aerobic Shape

If you have been recently following the workout described in my book *The Fat-Burning Workout*, you are ready to do this workout with no break-in period. *The Fat-Burning Workout* has put you in optimum weight-training and aerobic shape.

However, just to give yourself time to get used to the new method of working, I advise you to take advantage of all of the fifteen-second rests for at least the first week. After that you can go at your own pace.

If you have recently been following a weight-training workout such as the one I describe in *Cameo Fitness, Hard Bodies, The Hard Bodies Express Workout, Now or Never, Perfect Parts,* or *The 12-Minute Total-Body Workout,* or *Better and Better,* and in addition have been doing aerobic activities, such as running, step aerobics, bicycle riding, etc., you are in optimum weight-training and aerobic shape. But since you have never combined the two in a workout program, you may need a little break-in period—but then again, you may not. Therefore I will give you an option. You can try to do the workout as above—taking advantage of the fifteen-second rests for only the first week and then going at your own pace, or you can follow the advice in the next paragraph, for those who have been following a workout such as above but are not in aerobic shape.

Breaking In If You Have Already Been Working with Weights and Are Not in Aerobic Shape

If you have recently been following a weight-training workout such as the ones mentioned in the above paragraphs, but you have not been doing any aerobic activity, I want you to rest fifteen seconds between each and every exercise. Yes. I am telling you to commit the cardinal sin of cutting apart the Siamese twins—but only for one week, until you get used to the program. For the second week I want you to take advantage of the fifteen-second rests between intersets. After that you may go at your own pace.

Breaking In If You Are in Aerobic Shape, Are Basically Strong, but Have Little or No Experience in Working with Weights

Consider the first few weeks as a warm-up. Follow this modified plan, concentrating on learning the basic movement of the exercises.

Week 1: Do set 1 of each exercise. Rest fifteen seconds between each exercise. (You are committing the crime of breaking up the intersets only for this one week.)

Week 2: Do set 1 of each exercise, working in intersets (you are no longer breaking up the intersets). Take full advantage of the fifteen-second rest after each interset.

Week 3: Do all three sets of each interset. No rests between intersets. Take full advantage of the fifteen-second rests after each interset.

Week 4: You may go at your own pace.

Breaking In If You Have Never Worked with Weights, Are Not in Aerobic Shape, and Are Very Weak

Please don't be discouraged if this is you. You are my favorite client, because I get the greatest thrill in seeing how much progress you will make in a matter of months. What seems to be an insurmountable obstacle now, will appear to be a mere anthill to be stepped over if you are patient with yourself and give yourself some time to break in. You can do it. Easy does it, one step at a time. A journey of a thousand miles begins with a single step.

For the first two weeks, you will do the exercise movements without weight, but you will perform them in exactly the same manner as the full, regular workout.

Week 1: Do set 1—no weight. Do not break up the intersets (e.g., do a set of plié squats and standing back leg extensions without resting). Take full advantage of the fifteen-second rest between intersets.

Week 2: Do sets 1, 2, and 3—no weight. Do not break up the intersets. Take full advantage of the fifteen-second rests between intersets.

Week 3: Do set 1 only—one- to three-pound weight only. Rest fifteen seconds between each exercise (you're committing the cardinal sin of breaking up the intersets, but only for weeks 3, 4, and 5).

Week 4: Do sets 1 and 2—one- to three-pound weight only. Rest fifteen seconds between each exercise (you're committing the cardinal crime of breaking up the intersets, but only for this and one more week).

Week 5: Do sets 1, 2, and 3—one- to three-pound weight only. Rest fifteen seconds between each exercise (this is the last week you will commit the cardinal sin of breaking up the Siamese twins—the intersets).

Week 6: Do set 1 only—one- to three-pound weight only. Don't break up your intersets. Rest zero to fifteen seconds after each interset.

Week 7: Do sets 1 and 2—one- to three-pound weight only. Don't break up your intersets. Rest zero to fifteen seconds after each interset.

Week 8: Do sets 1, 2, and 3—one- to three-pound weight only. Don't break up your intersets. Rest zero to fifteen seconds after each interset. You are in the full program.

Week 9: You may go at your own pace, eliminating rests as you please. You are now free to raise your weights as your body becomes stronger.

Note: The term *weight* includes free weights and/or exercise machines.

THERAPEUTIC ALTERNATIVES

In the past I have gotten many letters from women who cannot do certain exercises because of back or knee problems. They have asked me to give them substitutes, and I have done so in this book. The therapeutic alternatives challenge the same muscle as the regular exercise, only they are easier on the knee or back, whatever the case may be. Of course, you should check with your doctor first. If he or she gives the OK, then simply do the therapeutic alternatives in place of the difficult exercise and follow the rest of the program exactly as written.

VARIATIONS

You may take advantage of the variations anytime you get bored with a given exercise.

STRETCHING

Before starting your workout, if you wish, you may do three repetitions of each exercise for the entire routine, without weight. However, since this program involves working with very light weights for the first set, you may not feel that stretching is necessary.

Some people enjoy a little stretching before a workout, not only to prepare the muscles for the workout but to prepare the mind as well. I am just the opposite of such people. Taking time to stretch is an annoyance to me. I am too impatient to waste time stretching. I'm also very busy and don't want to waste time with preliminaries unless it is absolutely necessary. Since the first set of each exercise is so light and provides a natural stretch, I say to myself, "Why bother?" But don't follow my lead unless you are so inclined.

THE GYM WORKOUT

If you choose to work out in a gym, you have two options: you can use the gym machines suggested in the individual exercise instructions, or you may pick and choose which exercises you want to do with free weights and which exercises you want to do with machines.

When I go to a gym, I usually use only a few machines and perform most of my exercises with a few pairs of dumbbells that I carry off into a corner, with a bench.

HOME OR GYM: WHICH IS BETTER?

Some of us don't have a choice. We are simply too busy to go to a gym. If we had to depend upon a gym workout, we would probably work out once a month. Others of us are private people—we feel self-conscious and don't want anyone looking at us as we sweat and groan.

Then there is the financial consideration. Think of all the money you can save by simply buying three sets of dumbbells and a bench! Gym memberships today range from a minimum of four hundred dollars a year up to two thousand—and even more. The exercise equipment will cost less than half of the lowest yearly gym membership and will last not for one year, but probably forever.

If we can save so much money by working at home, why do people go to gyms at all? In a gym you can enjoy the company of other people who are working out. In the presence of others, the time may seem to go faster. (But it will *actually* go more slowly if you fall into the trap of talking while you are working out!) You may feel comforted by the fact that you are not alone in your—shall I say "misery"? (Tongue in cheek of course, you will love the workout after a short time.)

I fall somewhere between the two categories. I usually don't have the time to go to a gym, so I do most of my work at home. But I am a gym member because at times I crave the camaraderie of fellow exercisers. I also like to take advantage of certain exercise machines, just for a change.

So do whatever pleases you. That's the beauty of this workout. There are no rules about where to work out. It's your decision completely.

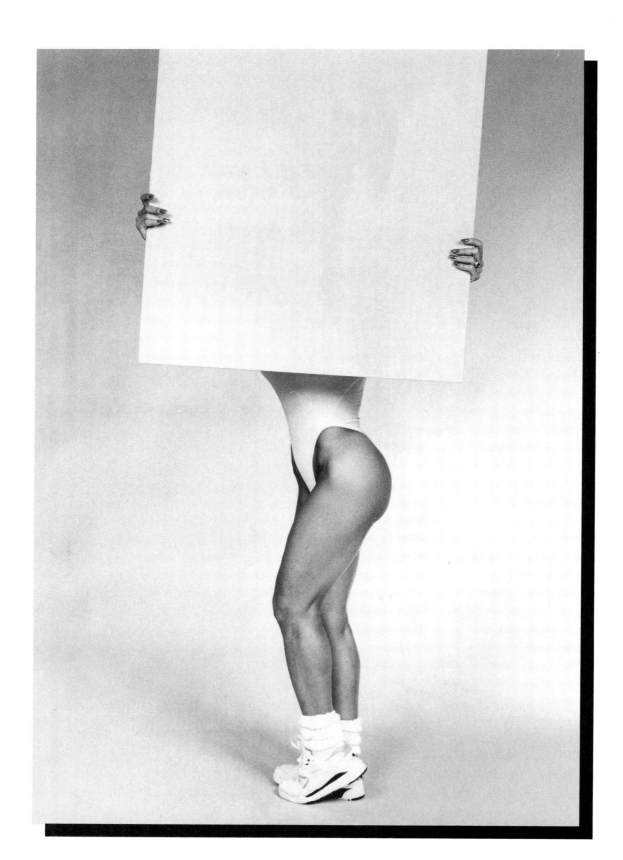

5

DAY ONE—
LOWER AND MIDDLE
BODY WORKOUT

Since it is our goal to get the body in shape from the bottom up and to attack head-on rather than avoid the previously dreaded lower and middle body areas, we will begin where it used to hurt—with the hips/buttocks, thighs, and abdominals. You will be delighted to find that exercising these previously dreaded body parts is no longer a horrific chore. The energy-efficient method of the interset has changed all of that, because as mentioned before, now you can rest one body part while exercising another; so even though you keep moving, you don't feel exhausted. In truth the lower and middle body workout will seem to be a relaxing proposition compared to previous routines you've done.

Before beginning the workout, quickly read the information on how to do the lower and middle body workout, and then once you are working out, go back, when necessary, to review. The information is given in order of the exercises: lower body is discussed first and then middle body.

THE LOWER BODY WORKOUT

You will be doing seven twin sets of exercises for the thighs and hips/buttocks. Those with knee or back problems may take advantage of an exercise's therapeutic alternative if the exercise itself would be too difficult.

THIGH–HIP/BUTTOCK INTERSETS

Thighs

1. Plié squat (*or* lying one-legged inner-thigh squeeze)

2. Bugs Bunny lunge (*or* standing one-legged thigh sweep)

3. Sissy squat (*or* modified sissy squat)

4. Leg extension

5. Hack squat (*or* toes-pointed-out leg extension)

6. Leg curl

7. Lying inner-thigh scissor

Hips/Buttocks

1. Standing back leg extension

2. Standing butt squeeze

3. Straight-leg kick-up

4. Vertical scissor

5. Feather kick-up

6. Prone butt lift

7. Lying butt lift

Note: Exercises in parentheses are therapeutic alternatives and may be used to replace the exercises they follow. These exercises have been provided for those who, due to back or knee problems, find the original exercise too difficult to perform.

How to Do the Lower Body Workout: Review

Do your first interset of the twin plié squat and the standing back leg extension without resting between sets. Rest zero to fifteen seconds, and then do a second set of that duet, again without breaking up the Siamese twins. Again, rest zero to fifteen seconds and complete your final twin set of that exercise combination. Now rest zero to fifteen seconds and move to your first interset of the next exercise combination, the Bugs Bunny lunge and the standing butt squeeze. Rest zero to fifteen seconds . . . and so on, until you have completed all seven twin sets—your entire thigh–hip/buttock routine. Then rest zero to fifteen seconds and begin your abdominal workout. Complete it in the same manner. (The abdominal workout will be discussed later in this chapter.) For a full review on how to do the Bottoms Up! Workout, see chapter 4.

Sets and Repetitions

You will do three sets of twelve to fifteen repetitions for all thigh exercises, and three sets of fifteen to twenty-five repetitions for all hip/buttock exercises. (Do the extra repetitions for the hip/buttock exercises whenever you feel that fifteen repetitions are not enough of a challenge. Your body will tell you.)

Note that you will be using weight for your thigh exercises, but not for your hip/buttock exercises, therefore, you will probably have the energy to do extra repetitions for your hip/buttock area.

Twelve to fifteen repetitions seem to be the ideal amount of challenge for those women who want to have firm thighs but who do not want to build any significant size in that area. If you do more than twelve to fifteen repetitions, you will wear down hard-earned thigh muscle, but if you go much below that number, you will not significantly challenge your thigh muscle (unless of course your goal is to put on size in that area, in which case you will be using heavy weights, doing less repetitions, and resting longer between sets. See page 81 for further information about putting on size).

Weights

You will need three sets of dumbbells for your thigh–hip/buttock workout: three-pound dumbbells, five-pound dumbbells, and eight-pound dumbbells. Later, as you get stronger, you will advance to fives, eights, and tens, and so on, until you are using, at most, tens, fifteens, and twenties (much later—maybe never).

For the thigh workout you will use the modified pyramid system, increasing the weights with each set, but you will never let your repetitions go below twelve to fifteen per set. This is a new concept. The usual method of pyramiding requires that you sacrifice at least two repetitions each time you raise the weight. In this case you may still sacrifice one repetition for each set if you so choose. (Instead of doing, say, fifteen repetitions for each set, you may want to do the following:

> **Set 1:** fifteen repetitions, three pounds
> **Set 2:** fourteen repetitions, five pounds
> **Set 3:** twelve to thirteen repetitions, eight pounds

Why do I insist that you never go below twelve to fifteen repetitions for thigh work? Experimentation has shown me that the best way to get maximum fat reduction and muscle tone on the thighs without bulk is to pyramid the weights but to keep the repetitions at twelve to fifteen for all sets.

No weight is used for the hip/buttock area because your goal is to tighten and tone that area while reducing its size.

REPS AND WEIGHTS FOR LOWER BODY WORKOUT

Thighs	**Hips/Buttocks**
Set 1: twelve to fifteen repetitions, three pounds	fifteen to twenty-five repetitions, no weight
Set 2: twelve to fifteen repetitions, five pounds	fifteen to twenty-five repetitions, no weight
Set 3: twelve to fifteen repetitions, eight pounds	fifteen to twenty-five repetitions, no weight

Raising the Weights As You Get Stronger

After working out for about three weeks, you may find that the weights you are using feel a bit too light. In other words, if you find yourself flying through the workout without a challenge, it's time to raise your overall weights. For example, if you were using dumbbells of three pounds, five pounds, and eight pounds, it may be time to advance to dumbbells of five pounds, eight pounds, and ten pounds.

After, say, another month, you may find that again, the weights have become too easy. Now you may want to raise the weights again.

The Plateau

Since this is a very intense workout, you cannot go extremely high in weight even if you want to. The highest weights you should ever use with this workout are dumbbells of ten, fifteen, and twenty pounds, unless of course you modify the workout as described below, in order to build larger muscles.

Sets and Repetitions for Building Larger Thigh Muscles

First of all, why would any woman want to build her thigh muscles? Some women like muscular thighs. They enjoy feeling strong, they believe they are appealing, and they have been encouraged by men who fully agree with them. Other women have no choice. They have dieted down and worked out, and now they have slim legs, but the skin of the thigh is loose, and it hangs over the knee. Whether this has happened because of aging or genetics, the only way to remedy the problem is to build up the muscle in the thigh area. You will know if this applies to you only after you have done the workout the regular way for about six months. (If at this time you realize that you must put on size, you will not have wasted six months. Your effort will have gone into tightening and toning of the thigh muscles. Now you will simply make them bigger.)

If you want to build your thigh muscles, you must use heavier weights, rest longer between twin sets (forty-five to sixty seconds), and use the true modified pyramid system (see below). You will of course keep your hip/buttock workout the same, using no weights and doing fifteen to twenty-five repetitions. Here's how your workout will look:

MODIFIED PYRAMID SYSTEM

Thighs	Hips/Buttocks
Set 1: twelve repetitions, ten pounds	fifteen to twenty-five repetitions, no weight
Rest 30-45 seconds	
Set 2: ten repetitions, fifteen pounds	fifteen to twenty-five repetitions, no weight
Rest 30-45 seconds	
Set 3: six to eight repetitions, twenty pounds	fifteen to twenty-five repetitions, no weight
Rest 30-45 seconds	

Use a barbell, plates, and a squat rack. An even better way to build your thigh muscles is to do barbell squats and lunges. For this you will need a barbell, some plates, and a squat rack.

If you are using a squat rack and a barbell, here is how your thigh workout will look:

Set 1: twelve repetitions, twenty-five pounds (barbell only)
Rest 30-45 seconds

Set 2: ten repetitions, thirty-five pounds (barbell and 2 five-pound plates)
Rest 30-45 seconds

Set 3: six to eight repetitions, forty-five pounds (barbell and 2 ten-pound plates)
Rest 30-45 seconds

Your goal will be to continue to add weight to your thigh routine as your thighs become stronger. Eventually, you may be using as much as 135 to 165 pounds for barbell squats.

As mentioned above, you will always keep the hip/buttock work the same. As you go along, you will want to keep adding weight to your thigh exercises until you are using at least a hundred pounds for your last set of six to eight repetitions. (See specific exercise instructions under "Alternate" for information on when to substitute a barbell for the dumbbells.)

THIGH–HIP/BUTTOCK ROUTINE

1. Plié Squat and Standing Back Leg Extension

Thighs: Plié Squat

Develops, shapes, and gives definition to the front thigh muscle (quadriceps), and especially tightens and tones the inner thigh.

STANCE: Hold a dumbbell in the center of your body with both hands, your arms straight down at the center of your body. Place your heels about six to eight inches apart with your toes pointed outward as far as possible. Keep your back erect and focus your eyes on a point in front of you.

MOVEMENT: Bending at the knees, descend to a nearly squatting position until your thighs are parallel to the floor. (If you cannot get that low, go as far as possible and stop, or use the therapeutic alternative to this exercise.) Feel the stretch in your inner thigh muscles and return to start. Flex your front and inner thigh muscles and repeat the movement until you have completed your set. Without resting, proceed to the other exercise in this twin set, the standing back leg extension.

ALERT: Be careful to keep your back straight. Do not lean forward or tip back. For maximum inner-thigh emphasis, remember to keep your toes pointed outward throughout the exercise.

VARIATION: You may perform this exercise with a barbell placed on your shoulders, and with your toes pointed out or nearly straight ahead (the straight-ahead position puts a greater emphasis on your front thigh muscle).

GYM WORKOUT: You may perform this exercise on any squat machine, with toes pointed out or toes pointed straight ahead.

Start

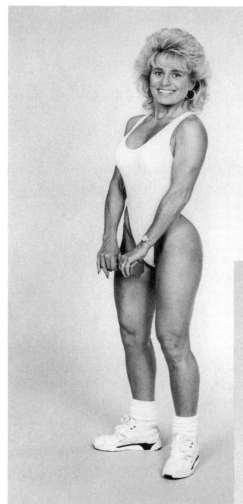

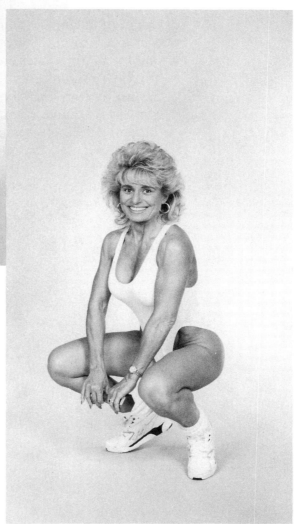

Finish

Therapeutic Alternative to the Plié Squat: Lying One-Legged Inner-Thigh Squeeze

Tightens, tones, and defines the inner thigh area, and helps to tighten the hip/buttock area.

STANCE: Lie on the floor flat on your back with your shoulders off the floor. Extend your legs straight out in front of you, heels about six inches apart, and lock your knees.

MOVEMENT: Raise your right heel six inches off the floor, and keeping your right knee locked, bring your right heel toward your left ankle. Continue moving in this direction, at the same time squeezing your right buttock and inner thigh, until your right heel crosses over your left ankle. Keeping the pressure on your right buttock and inner thigh, return to start position and repeat the movement until you have completed your set. Complete the set for the other leg. Without resting, proceed to the other exercise in this twin set, the standing back leg extension.

ALERT: Do not bend at the knee. Keep your leg extended fully. Keep the pressure on your buttock and inner thigh throughout the movement. (Keeping pressure on the buttock helps to keep pressure on the inner thigh as well.)

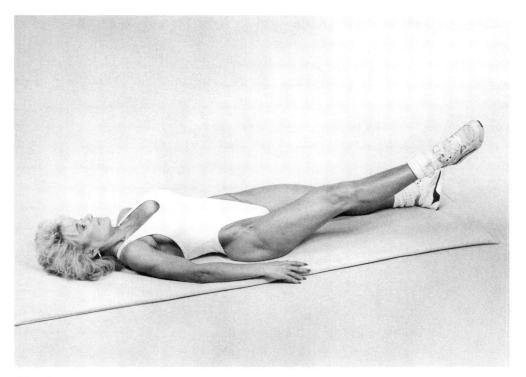

Start

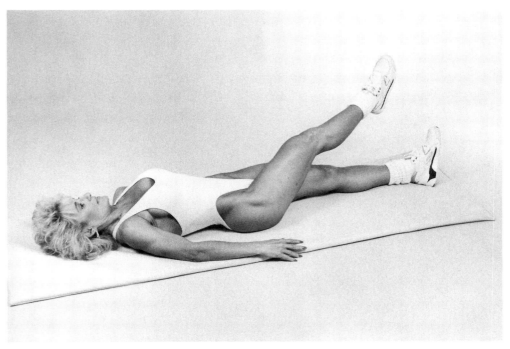

Finish

Hips/Buttocks: Standing Back Leg Extension

Tightens and tones the entire hip-buttock and helps to remove "saddle bags."

STANCE: Facing an object you can use for support, stand with your back straight and your feet shoulder width apart. If necessary, grasp the object as you work.

MOVEMENT: With toes pointed behind you, extend your left leg about eight inches behind you while at the same time squeezing your left buttock as hard as possible. Keeping the pressure on your buttock, return to start position and repeat the movement until you have completed your set. Repeat the set for your other leg. Rest zero to fifteen seconds and do a second set of the plié squat and the standing back leg extension. (You will do three sets of this exercise combination in all and then proceed to the next thigh–hip/buttock twin, the Bugs Bunny lunge and the standing butt squeeze.)

Remember, you will be doing twelve to fifteen repetitions for each thigh exercise, and fifteen to twenty-five repetitions for each hip/buttock exercise.

ALERT: Keep the pressure on your working buttock. Squeeze as hard as possible. Do not hold your breath. Breathe naturally.

VARIATION: You may perform this movement kneeling. You will then extend only your waist-to-knee area behind you.

GYM WORKOUT: You may substitute this exercise for any exercise done on a hip/buttock machine.

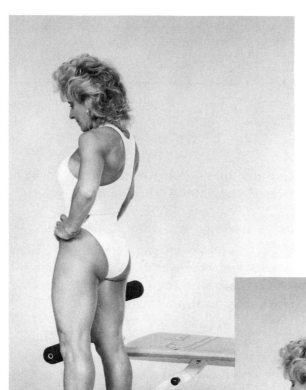

Start

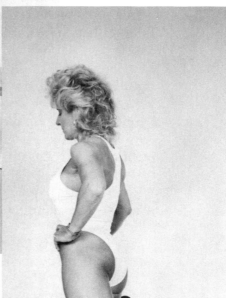

Finish

2. Bugs Bunny Lunge and Standing Butt Squeeze

Thighs: Bugs Bunny Lunge

Tightens, tones, and defines the inner thigh, helps to develop the front thigh muscle (quadriceps), and helps to remove "saddle bags."

STANCE: Stand with your feet a natural width apart. Keep your back back straight. Hold a dumbbell in each hand, palms facing your body, and arms straight down at your sides. Look at a point directly in front of you.

MOVEMENT: Keeping your left foot in place, and with the toes of your right leg pointed out as far as possible, lunge forward with your right leg about two and a half feet. You will be bending your right knee as you lunge. Flex your left leg and feel the stretch in your lunging leg. Return to start position and repeat the movement until you have completed your set. Repeat the set for your other leg. Without resting, proceed to the other exercise in this twin set, the standing butt squeeze.

ALERT: Keeping the toes of your lunging leg pointed out will at first seem to be a very awkward proposition. In time, however, you will get used to it and may even enjoy it. It's well worth the effort because this exercise really helps to tighten the inner thigh and places pretty lines of definition in that area.

VARIATION: You may do barbell lunges by placing a barbell on your shoulders. You may do regular lunges by keeping your toes pointed straight ahead (this method places a greater emphasis on the front thigh muscle).

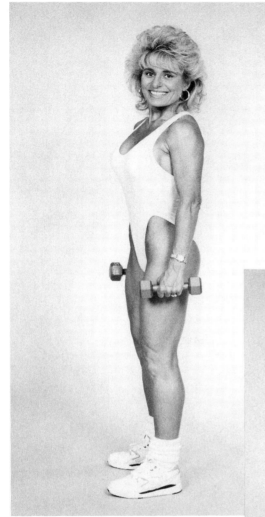

Start

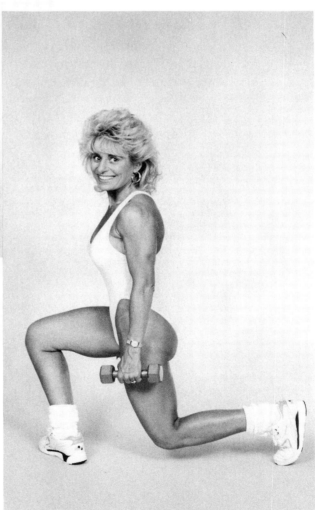

Finish

Therapeutic Alternative to the Bugs Bunny Lunge: Standing One-Legged Thigh Sweep

Tightens and tones the entire inner thigh area. Helps to tighten and lift the hip/buttock area.

STANCE: Stand with your feet a natural width apart and with your back erect. With your knee locked and your toes pointed out in front of you, extend your right leg forward about six inches.

MOVEMENT: Keeping your knee locked and flexing your right inner thigh as hard as possible, sweep your right leg toward your left toes, continue the movement until your right heel crosses over your left toes. Keeping the pressure on your right inner thigh, return to start position and repeat the movement until you have completed your set. Repeat the set for your other leg. Without resting, proceed to the other exercise in this twin set, the standing butt squeeze.

ALERT: Don't bend the knee of your working leg. Keep it locked or you will take pressure off the inner thigh muscle. Don't hold your breath. Breathe naturally.

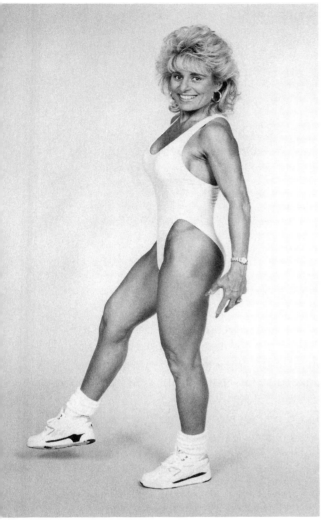

Start

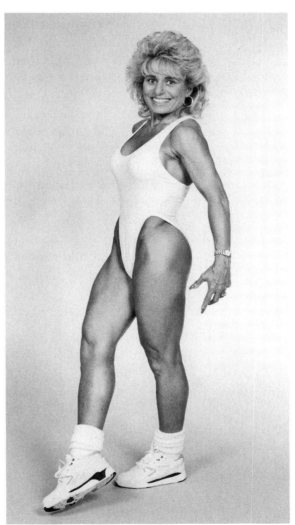

Finish

Hips/Buttocks: Standing Butt Squeeze

94

Tightens and tones the entire hip/buttock area.

STANCE: Stand with your feet a natural width apart and with your back erect. Hold a dumbbell in each hand, palms facing your body. Lower your body about four inches by bending at the knee.

MOVEMENT: Flex your entire hip/buttock area as hard as possible, and rise until your knees are nearly locked, thrusting your hips slightly forward as you rise. Keeping the pressure on your hip/buttock area, as you go. Return to start and repeat the movement until you have completed your set. Rest zero to fifteen seconds and do a second set of the Bugs Bunny lunge and the standing butt squeeze. (You will do three sets of this exercise combination in all and then proceed to the next thigh–hip/buttock combination, the sissy squat and the straight-leg kick-up.)

Remember, you will be doing twelve to fifteen repetitions for each thigh exercise, and fifteen to twenty-five repetitions of each hip/buttock exercise.

ALERT: This exercise seems awkward at first, but once you get used to it and really begin to flex your buttocks, you will find it quite enjoyable.

VARIATION: You may do this exercise with a barbell placed over your shoulders.

GYM WORKOUT: You may substitute this exercise for any exercise done on a hip/buttock machine.

Start

Finish

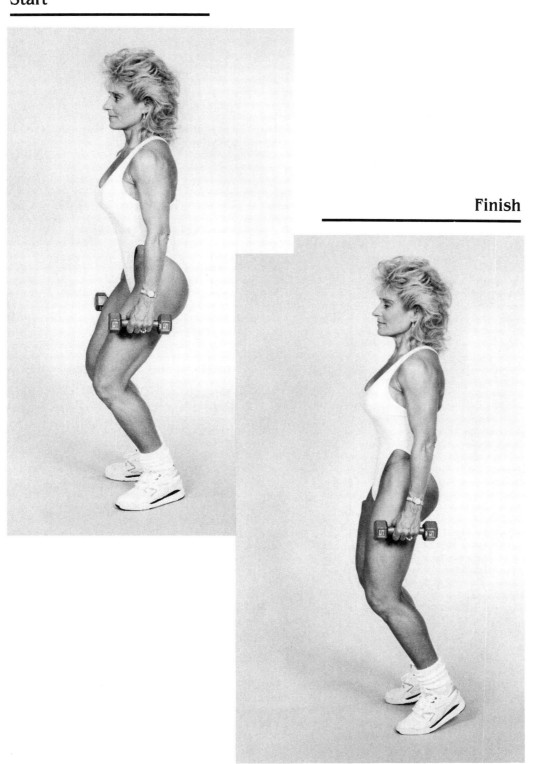

3. Sissy Squat and Straight-Leg Kick-Up

Thighs: Sissy Squat

Tightens, tones, and defines the front thigh muscle (quadriceps), tightens the back thigh muscle (biceps femoris, or hamstrings), and gives definition to the inner thigh. Helps to tighten the hip/buttock area.

STANCE: Stand with your feet about five inches apart and your toes pointed slightly outward. Place your right hand on a stable object, such as a table, bar, or railing.

MOVEMENT: Flexing your front and inner thigh muscles as hard as possible, raise yourself up on your toes. At the same time lean your upper body back as far as you can go, and squeeze your buttocks as hard as possible. You will be completely up on your bent toes at this point and you will feel an extreme stretch in your front thigh muscles. Keep your hips in line with your ankles as you work. Continue to keep the pressure on your front thigh muscles and return to start position, repeating the movement until you have completed your set. Without resting, proceed to the other exercise in this twin set, the straight-leg kick-up.

ALERT: Do not be discouraged by the seeming awkwardness of this exercise. It is very effective. If the instructions are difficult to follow, look at the photographs and try to copy what you see.

GYM WORKOUT: You may perform this exercise with a weighted belt (used by bodybuilders).

Therapeutic Alternative to the Sissy Squat

You may perform the squat by descending only partially—as far as your knees will allow. If you flex your quadriceps (front thigh) muscles as you work, you will still get a lot out of the exercise.

Start

Finish

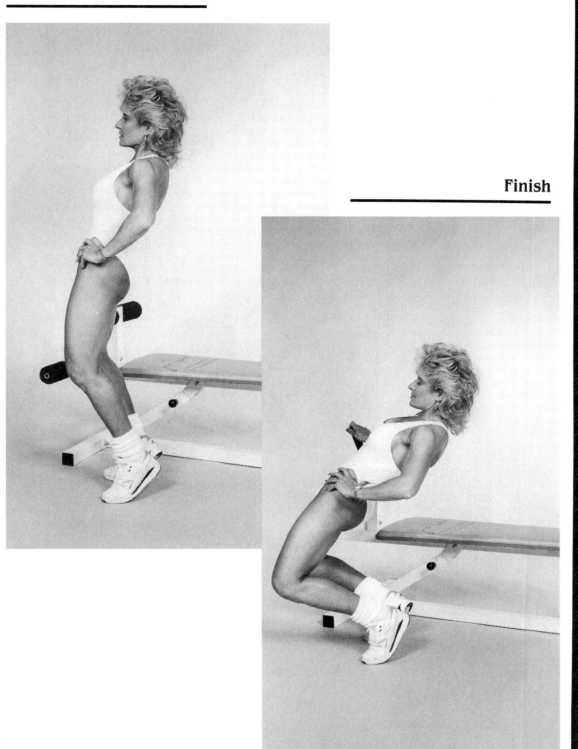

Hips/Buttocks: Straight-Leg Kick-Up

Tightens, tones, and lifts the entire hip/buttock area, and helps to remove "saddle bags."

STANCE: Get into an all-fours position on the floor. With your toes flexed back, extend your left leg straight out behind you, in line with your body, your toes touching the floor.

MOVEMENT: Squeezing your right buttock as hard as possible and keeping your right knee locked and your leg in line with your body as much as possible, raise your left leg behind you as high as you can. Flex your left buttocks and return to start position. Repeat the movement until you have completed your set. Perform the exercise for the other side of your body. Rest zero to fifteen seconds and do a second set of the sissy squat and the straight-leg kick-up. (You will do three sets of this exercise combination and then proceed to the next thigh–hip/buttock combination, the leg extension and the vertical scissor.)

Remember, you will be doing twelve to fifteen repetitions for each thigh exercise, and fifteen to twenty-five repetitions of each hip/buttock exercise.

ALERT: Remember to squeeze your working buttock through the exercise. In order to see how effective the exercise is, place your hand on the working buttock as you go.

GYM WORKOUT: You may substitute this exercise for any exercise done on a hip/buttock machine.

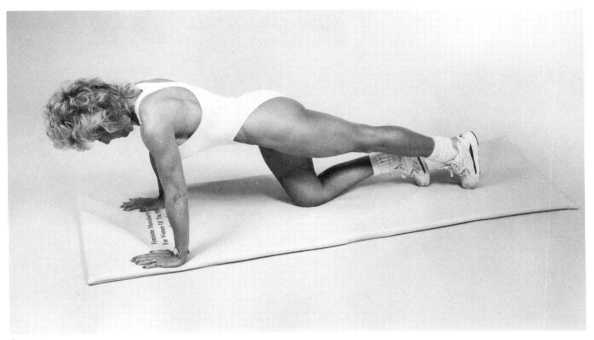

Start

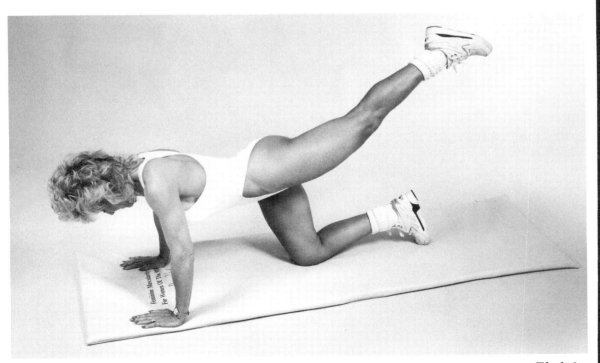

Finish

4. Leg Extension and Vertical Scissor

Thighs: Leg Extension

Tightens, tones, and strengthens the front thigh muscle (quadriceps).

STANCE: Sit at the edge of a flat exercise bench or chair with a dumbbell held between your ankles. Your knees should be bent, and your legs should be in an L position.

MOVEMENT: Holding the dumbbell securely between your ankles and flexing your front thigh muscles as hard as possible, extend your legs until they are straight out in front of you. Return to start position, and repeat the movement until you have completed your set.

ALERT: Do not jerk the weight up or let it nearly drop to the down position. Maintain control of your movements at all times. Do not hold your breath. Breathe naturally.

VARIATION: You may perform this exercise with your toes pointed out. This will place greater emphasis on your inner thigh area.

GYM WORKOUT: You may perform this exercise on any leg extension machine.

Start

Finish

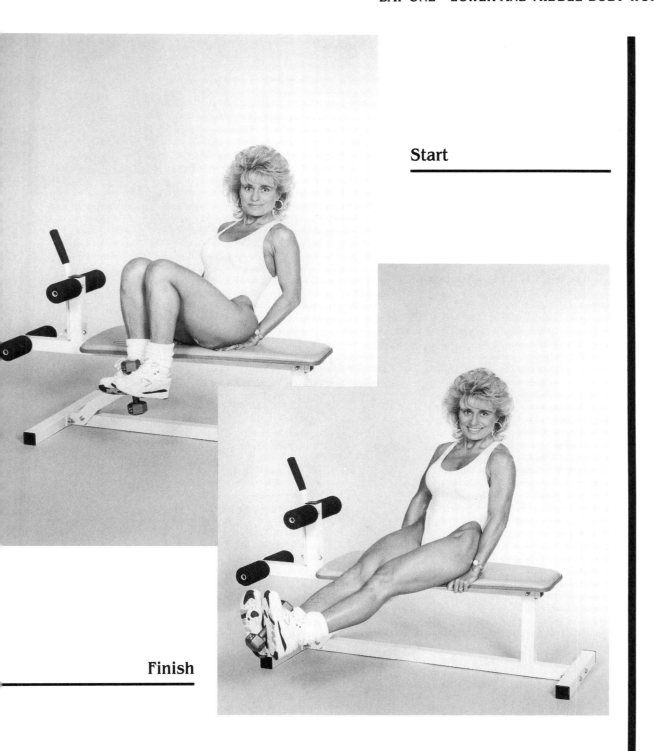

Hips/Buttocks: Vertical Scissor

Tightens and tones the outer and upper hip/buttock area. Also helps to firm the front thigh muscle (quadriceps).

STANCE: Sit at the edge of a flat exercise bench and place a hand, palm facing down, under each buttock. Extend your legs straight out in front of you until your knees are locked. Place your ankles about four inches apart. Point your toes forward.

MOVEMENT: Squeezing your hip/buttock area as hard as possible, scissor your legs up and down about twelve inches high each time. Continue this up and down movement until you have completed your set. Rest zero to fifteen seconds and do a second set of the leg extension and the vertical scissor. (You will do three sets of this exercise combination in all and then proceed to the next thigh– hip/buttock combination, the hack squat and the feather kick-up.)

Remember, you will be doing twelve to fifteen repetitions for each thigh exercise, and fifteen to twenty-five repetitions for each hip/buttock exercise.

ALERT: You may perform this exercise rapidly. As long as you keep the pressure on your hip/buttock area as you work, speed will not detract from the efficacy of the workout.

VARIATION: You may perform this exercise by scissoring your legs out and together. If you choose to do this, do not cross your legs one over the other on the in position; instead, let your ankles touch each time and scissor out as wide as possible.

GYM WORKOUT: You may substitute this exercise for any exercise performed on a hip/buttock machine.

Start

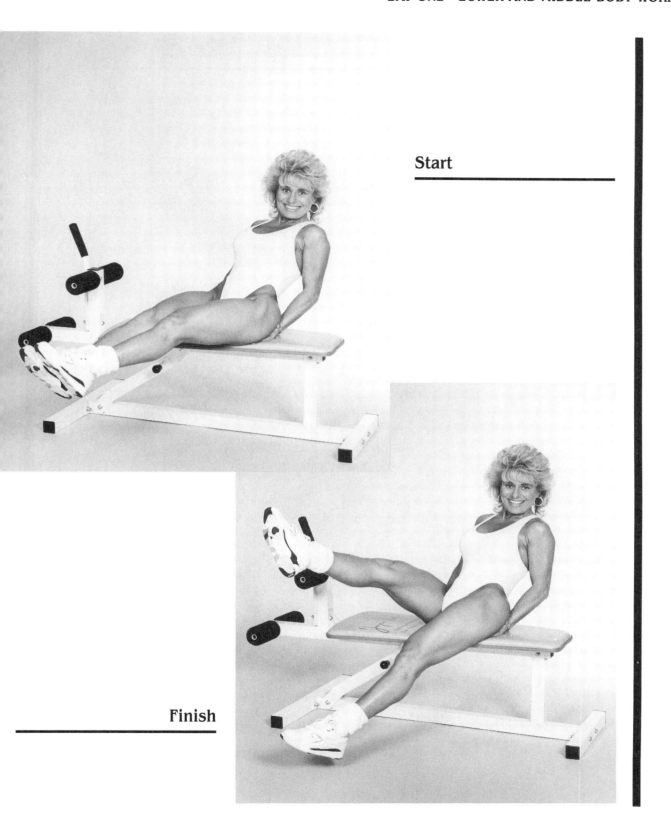

Finish

5. Hack Squat and Feather Kick-Up

Thighs: Hack Squat

Tightens, tones, and defines the entire front thigh muscle (quadriceps), helps to develop and tone the back thigh muscle (biceps femoris, or hamstrings), and helps to remove "saddle bags."

STANCE: Stand with your feet a natural width apart. Hold a dumbbell in each hand behind your back, palms facing away from your body, dumbbells in line with the back thighs.

MOVEMENT: Flexing your front and back thigh muscles as hard as possible, bend at the knee into a squatting position while at the same time letting the dumbbells descend in line with your back thighs. When your thighs are approximately parallel to the floor, return to start position and flex your front and back thigh muscles an extra pinch. Without resting, return to start position and repeat the movement until you have completed your set.

ALERT: You may rise slightly up on your toes as you descend in order to keep your balance. Remember to keep the dumbbells in line with your back thigh muscles as you descend to the squatting position.

GYM WORKOUT: You may perform this exercise on any hack squat machine.

Therapeutic Alternative to the Hack Squat

You may substitute the toes-pointed-out leg extension for this exercise (see the variation for the leg extension, page 88).

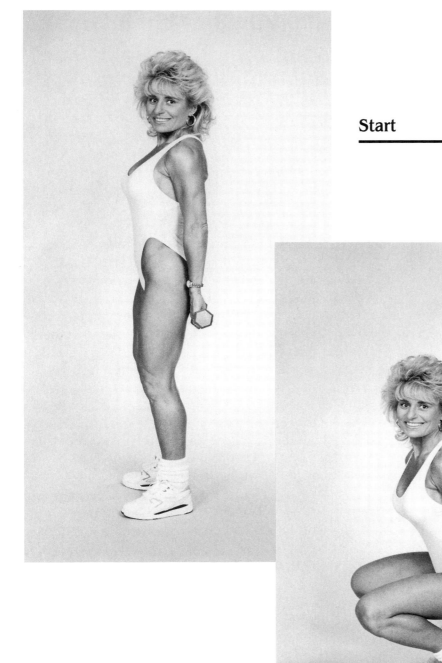

Start

Finish

Hips/Buttocks: Feather Kick-Up

Tightens and tones the entire hip/buttock area. Helps to firm the back thigh muscle (biceps femoris, or hamstrings), and helps to remove "saddle bags."

STANCE: Place yourself in an all-fours position on the floor. Raise your left thigh up and bend at the knee so that your leg takes the shape of an L.

MOVEMENT: Pointing your toes behind you, straighten your left leg by raising your leg and unbending your knee at the same time. Continue this movement until your knee is no longer bent and you cannot raise your leg any higher. Return to start position and repeat the movement until you have completed your set. Repeat the set for the other leg. Rest zero to fifteen seconds and do a second set of the hack squat and the feather kick-up. (You will do three sets of this exercise combination in all and then proceed to the next thigh–hip/buttock twin, the leg curl and the prone butt lift.)

Remember, you will be doing twelve to fifteen repetitions for each thigh exercise, and fifteen to twenty-five repetitions for each hip/buttock exercise.

ALERT: It is mandatory that you return to the L position each time you unbend your leg. This exercise is at first awkward, but once you get used to it, you will come to enjoy it. It is most effective!

GYM WORKOUT: This is the one hip/buttock exercise that may not be substituted for an exercise performed on a gym hip/buttock machine.

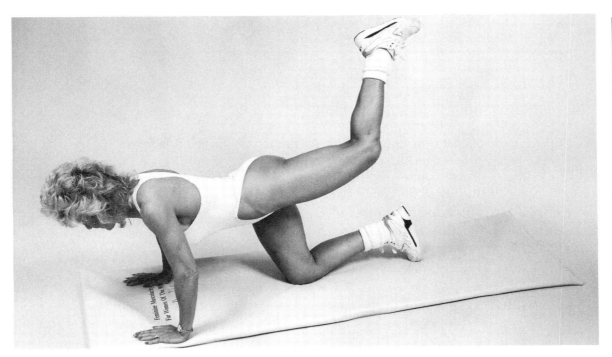

Start

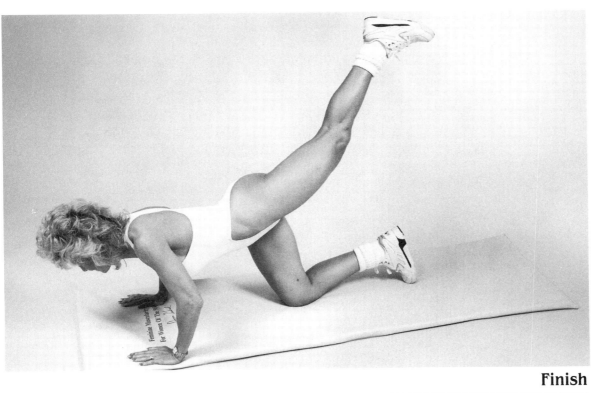

Finish

6. The Leg Curl and the Prone Butt Lift

Thighs: Leg Curl

Tightens, tones, and shapes the back thigh muscle (biceps femoris, or hamstrings).

STANCE: With a dumbbell placed between your feet, lie in a prone position on the floor or a flat exercise bench. Extend your legs straight out behind you and lean on your elbows for support.

MOVEMENT: Bending at the knees and flexing your back thigh muscles as hard as possible, raise your lower legs until they are perpendicular to the floor. Keeping the pressure on your back thigh muscles, return to start position and repeat the movement until you have completed your set. Without resting, proceed to the other exercise in this twin set, the prone butt lift.

ALERT: Be aware of the temptation to swing the dumbbell up and down. Keep your movements deliberate by constantly flexing your working back thigh muscles. If you squeeze your ankles together, you will accomplish two things at once: the dumbbell will remain stable as you work, and you will achieve a greater flex for your back thigh muscles.

GYM WORKOUT: You may perform this exercise on any gym leg-curl machine.

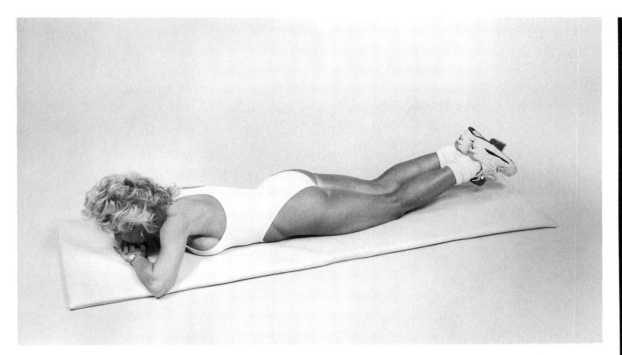

Start

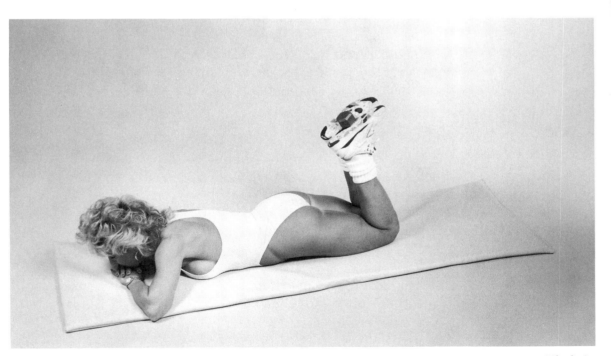

Finish

Hips/Buttocks: Prone Butt Lift

Tightens and tones the entire hip/buttock area, and helps to shape the back thigh muscle (biceps femoris, or hamstrings), and helps to remove "saddle bags." Strengthens the lower back.

STANCE: Lie on the floor on your stomach. Lean on your elbows for support. Extend your toes behind you. Your feet should be about twelve inches apart.

MOVEMENT: Squeezing your entire hip/buttock area as hard as possible and keeping your knees locked, lift both legs at once until you cannot go any higher. Your legs will naturally go into a wider position at this point (about eighteen inches apart). Continuing to keep the pressure on your hip/buttock area, return to start position and repeat the movement until you have completed your set. Rest zero to fifteen seconds and do a second set of the leg curl and prone butt lift. (You will do three sets of this exercise combination in all and then proceed to the last thigh–hip/buttock twin, the lying inner-thigh scissor and the lying butt lift.)

Remember, you will be doing twelve to fifteen repetitions for each thigh exercise, and fifteen to twenty-five repetitions for each hip/buttock exercise.

ALERT: Beware of the temptation to tense your lower back. Consciously relax your back as you work. You may want to keep your fingertips on your buttocks as you move in order to ensure that you are flexing that area to the fullest extent.

VARIATION: You may perform this exercise one leg at a time.

GYM WORKOUT: You may substitute this exercise for any exercise performed on a hip/buttock machine.

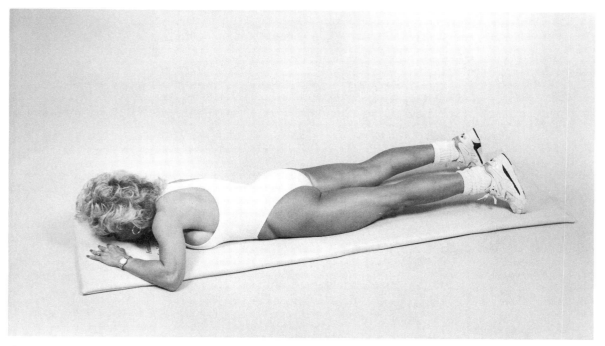

Start

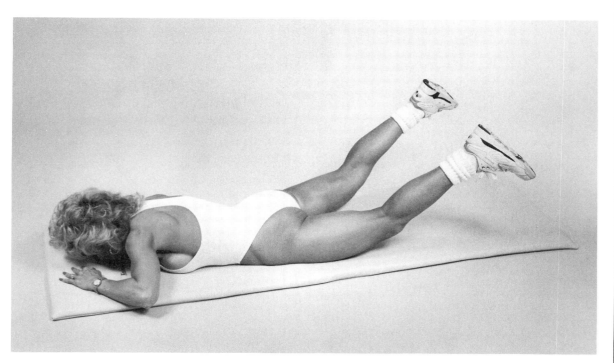

Finish

7. Lying Inner-Thigh Scissor and Lying Butt Lift

Thighs: Lying Inner-Thigh Scissor

Tightens, tones, and defines the entire inner thigh area. Helps to tighten and tone the entire hip/buttock area.

STANCE: Lie on the floor flat on your back (or with your shoulders off the floor) and your legs extended straight out in front of you. Point your toes out as far as possible, and touch your heels together.

MOVEMENT: Keeping your toes pointed out as far as possible, and with the pressure on your inner thighs, scissor your legs apart as wide as possible. Without resting, return to start position and repeat the movement until you have completed your set. Without resting, proceed to the other exercise in this twin set, the lying butt lift.

ALERT: Keep your knees locked and your toes pointed out throughout the movement. Scissor your legs only to the heel-to-heel position. Do not let your ankles cross each other. Don't hold your breath. Breathe naturally.

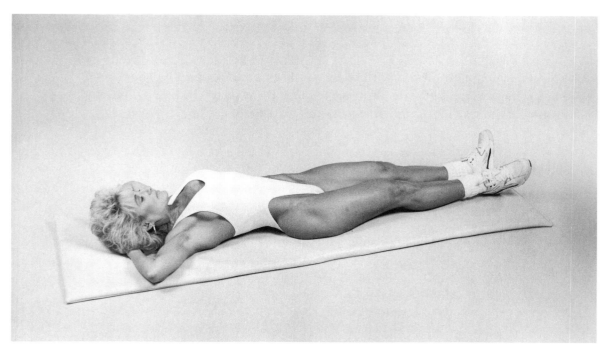

Start

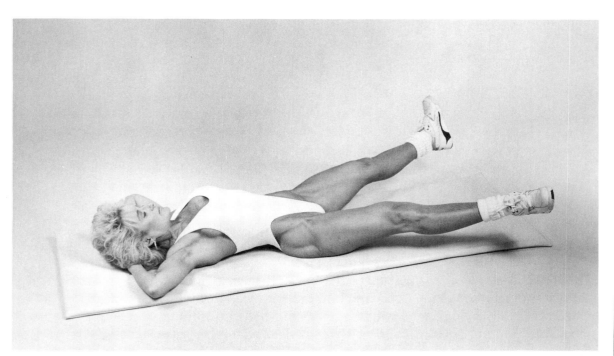

Finish

Hips/Buttocks: Lying Butt Lift

Tightens, tones, and lifts the entire hip/buttock area, and helps to remove "saddle bags." Strengthens and tones the back thigh muscle (biceps femoris, or hamstrings) and lower back area.

STANCE: Lie flat on your back on the floor and bend your knees until your feet are about eighteen inches apart and flat on the floor. Place a hand, palm up, under each buttock.

MOVEMENT: Squeezing your entire hip/buttock area as hard as possible, raise your pelvis to the highest position possible. Keeping the pressure on the hip/buttock area, return to start position and repeat the movement until you have completed your set. Rest zero to fifteen seconds and do a second set of the lying inner-thigh scissor and the lying butt lift. (You will do three sets of this exercise combination in all and then proceed to the abdominal workout.)

Remember, you will be doing twelve to fifteen repetitions for each thigh exercise, and fifteen to twenty-five repetitions for each hip/buttock exercise.

ALERT: Remember to flex your entire buttocks area throughout your exercise. Do not rest between repetitions. Keep up the pace.

GYM WORKOUT: You may substitute this exercise for any exercise performed on a hip/buttock machine.

Note: If you work out in a gym and choose to substitute the hip/buttock exercises for those done on hip/buttock machines, be sure to use only one machine exercise as a substitute for one exercise in this program. In other words, there are seven hip/buttock exercises in this workout, and unless you can find seven different exercises to perform on gym hip/buttock machines, you must do at least some of the hip/buttock exercises as described here. If you are working out in a gym, simply do them on the floor in any convenient area.

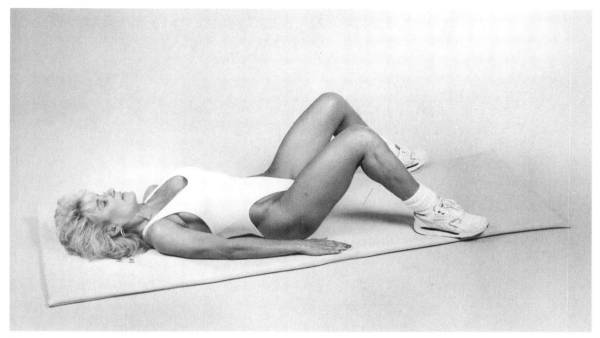

Start

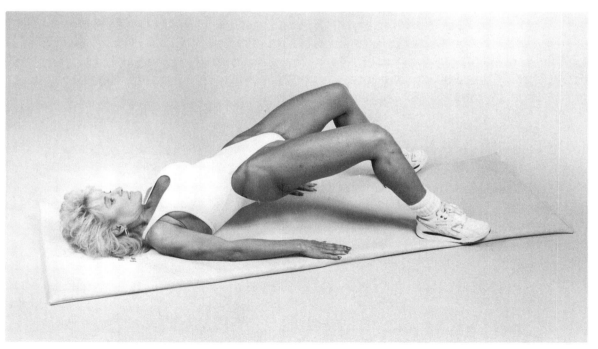

Finish

MIDDLE BODY WORKOUT: LOWER AND UPPER ABDOMINALS

You will work in exactly the same manner as above, doing one set of each of the twin pairs before you rest for zero to fifteen seconds.

Sets and Repetitions

You will do three sets of fifteen to twenty-five repetitions of each abdominal exercise.

Weights

No weights are needed for the abdominal workout, although they are optional. (See individual exercise instructions.)

There are five exercises for the abdominal area, and one optional exercise, making two twin sets and a single, or three twin sets. I suggest that you do the optional exercise for two reasons: it makes for a neat closure of the last, lonely nontwin, and it is so easy to incorporate as the position fits neatly with its partner. (You'll see.)

LOWER AND UPPER ABDOMINAL INTERSETS

Lower Abdominals

1. Knee-in (*or* reverse crunch)

2. Bent-knee leg raise (*or* six-inch leg raise)

Upper Abdominals

1. Crunch

2. Bent-knee sit-up (*or* knee-raised crunch)

Side Abdominals (Obliques)

1. Oblique crunch

2. Reverse crunch (*optional*)

Note: Exercises in parentheses are therapeutic alternatives and can be used as substitutes by those who have back problems. If you use the reverse crunch as a therapeutic alternative to the knee-in, you may repeat it again as a partner for the lonely oblique crunch. Don't worry that you will have done the same exercise twice. It's OK!

ABDOMINAL ROUTINE

1. Knee-in and Crunch

Lower Abdominals: Knee-in

Tightens and tones the entire lower abdominal area. Strengthens the lower back.

STANCE: Lie on the floor or on a mat. Extend your legs straight out in front of you. The small of your back should remain nearly flat to the floor.

MOVEMENT: Flexing your lower abdominal muscles as hard as possible and keeping your knees together, pull your knees in toward your chest until you cannot go any farther. Keeping the tension on your lower abdominal muscles, return to start position and repeat the movement until you have completed your set. Without resting, proceed to the other twin in this set, the crunch.

ALERT: It will be tempting to let your knees spread apart while you are exercising. This takes some of the tension off your lower abdominal area and makes the exercise less effective. Keep your knees together.

VARIATION: You may perform this exercise sitting at the edge of an exercise bench and holding onto the sides. If you lean back to a 30-degree angle and extend your legs straight out in front of you, you will be in a perfect exercise position.

WEIGHTS: You may perform this exercise with a three- to five-pound dumbbell held between your ankles.

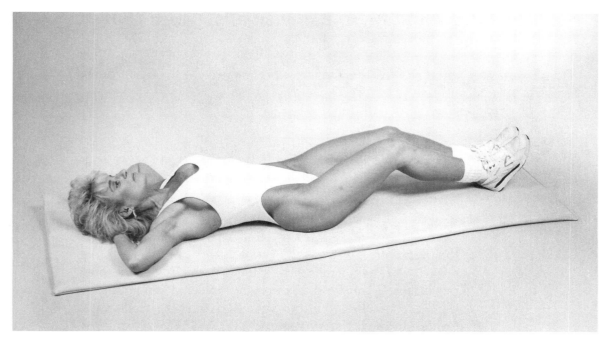

Start

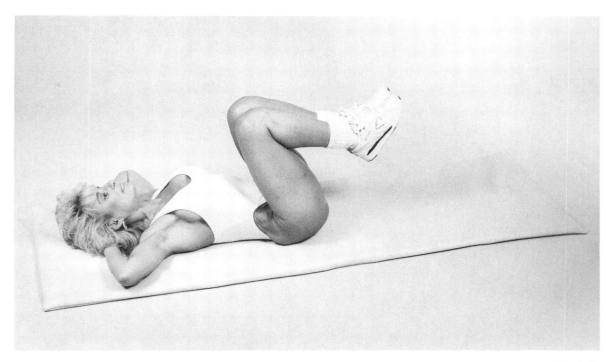

Finish

Therapeutic Alternative to the Knee-in: Reverse Crunch

Tightens, tones, and develops the lower abdominal area. Also strengthens the lower back muscles.

STANCE: Lie on the floor flat on your back with your knees completely bent (to an approximate 90-degree angle). You may place your hands at your sides, behind your head, or under your buttocks for support. Point your knees toward the ceiling.

MOVEMENT: Keeping your knees together, raise your lower abdominal area by bringing your knees as close to your chest as possible, all the time flexing your lower abdominals as hard as possible. Without resting, return to start position and repeat the movement until you have completed your set. Without resting, proceed to the other exercise in this twin set, the crunch.

ALERT: Beware of the temptation to bounce off the floor and to give yourself momentum to rock back and forth. Instead, maintain full control of your movements. Make each repetition deliberate.

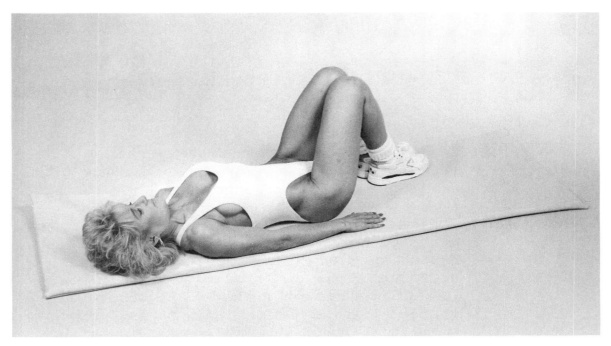

Start

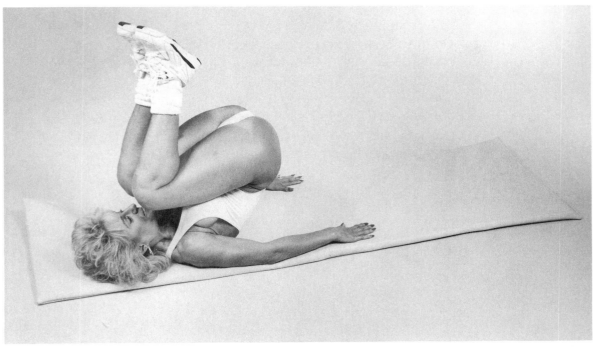

Finish

Upper Abdominals: Crunch

Tightens and tones the entire upper abdominal area. Helps to strengthen the lower back.

STANCE: Lie flat on your back on the floor, and bend your knees until the soles of your feet are flat on the ground. Place your hands behind your head or on your stomach.

MOVEMENT: Curl your body upward until only your shoulders are completely off the ground, all the time flexing your upper abdominal muscles as hard as possible. Without letting up on the tension, return to start position and repeat the movement until you have finished your set. Rest zero to fifteen seconds, and do a second set of the knee-in and the crunch. (You will do three sets of this exercise combination in all and then proceed to the next abdominal combination, the bent-knee leg raise and the bent-knee sit-up.)

Remember, you will do three sets of fifteen to twenty-five repetitions for each abdominal exercise.

ALERT: Do not rise to a sitting position. This is a crunch, not a sit-up. Rise only to shoulders-off-the-ground level.

VARIATION: You may perform the "crunch twist" by alternately twisting your body to each side as you crunch. You may perform this exercise by placing your legs over a flat exercise bench and crossing your legs at the ankles.

GYM WORKOUT: You may perform this exercise on any crunch machine.

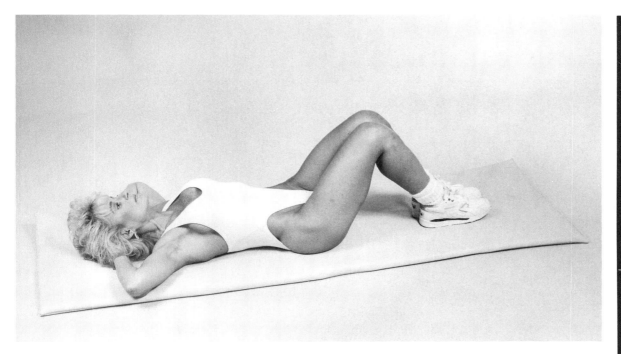

Start

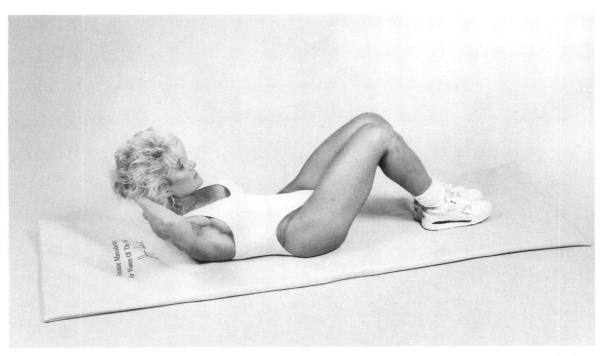

Finish

2. Bent-Knee Leg Raise and Bent-Knee Sit-Up

Lower Abdominals: Bent-Knee Leg-Raise

Tightens and tones the entire lower abdominal area. Helps to strengthen the lower back.

STANCE: Lie flat on your back on the floor or a bench with your hands at your sides, behind your head, or holding the sides of the bench. With your heels on the floor, bend your legs to nearly an L position. Keep your shoulders on the floor or bench.

MOVEMENT: Flexing your lower abdominal muscles as hard as possible, raise your legs (keeping them in the near-L position) until your thighs are a little higher than perpendicular to the floor. Continuing to keep the pressure on your lower abdominal muscles, return to start position and repeat the movement until you have completed your set. Without resting, proceed to the other exercise in this twin set, the bent-knee sit-up.

ALERT: Be careful not to arch your back. Keep your knees and ankles together throughout the movement.

WEIGHTS: You may perform this exercise with a three- to five-pound dumbbell between your ankles.

GYM WORKOUT: You may perform this exercise on any Roman chair by extending your legs out until they are parallel to the floor.

Therapeutic Alternative to the Leg Raise: Six-Inch Leg Raise

You may perform the bent-knee leg raise in the same manner as above, only instead of raising your legs until your thighs are perpendicular to the floor, raise them until the soles of your feet are only six inches off the

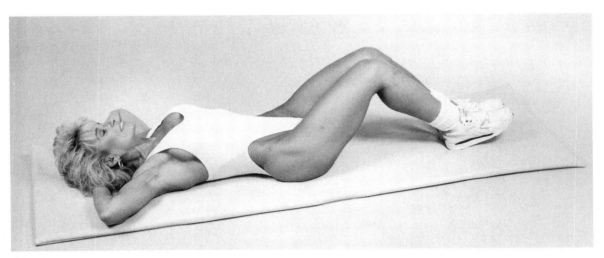

Start

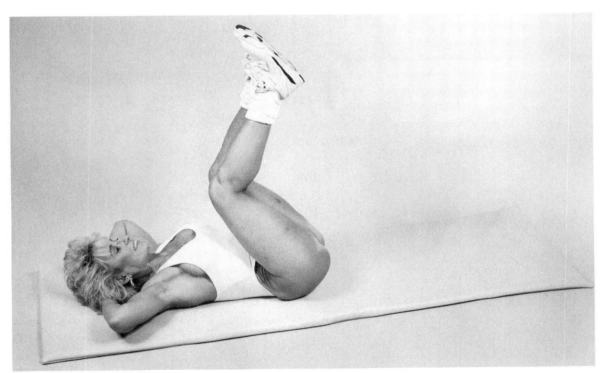

Finish

ground. You will still achieve a great deal of emphasis on the lower abdominal area, and you will have completely taken the pressure off your lower back.

Upper Abdominals: Bent-Knee Sit-Up

Tightens and tones the upper abdominal area. Helps to strengthen the lower back.

STANCE: Lie flat on your back on the floor, and bend your knees just until the soles of your feet are flat on the ground. Place your hands behind your head or cross them in front of you on your chest.

MOVEMENT: Flexing your upper abdominal muscles as hard as possible, raise yourself off the floor until you are sitting up. Your back should be nearly perpendicular to the floor. (The movement is one of curling rather than jerking.) Keeping the pressure on your upper abdominal muscles, return to start position and repeat the movement until you have completed your set. Rest zero to fifteen seconds, and do a second set of the bent-knee leg-raise and the bent-knee sit-up. (You will do three sets of this exercise combination in all and then proceed to the next exercise, the oblique crunch and, if you choose the option, the reverse crunch).

ALERT: In order to keep the strain off your back, be sure to keep your knees bent throughout the movement. Do not bounce off the floor. Maintain a fluid movement.

GYM WORKOUT: You may perform this exercise on any sit-up machine.

WEIGHTS: You may perform this exercise with a three- to ten-pound dumbbell or plate held on your upper abdominal area.

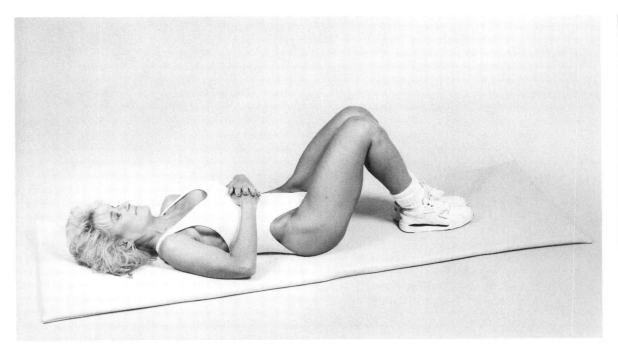

Start

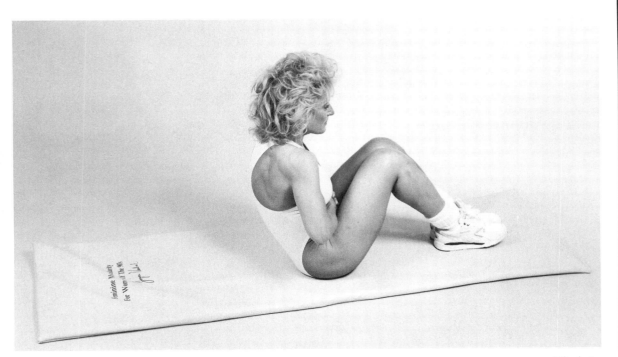

Finish

Therapeutic Alternative to the Bent-Knee Sit-up: Knee-Raised Crunch

Strengthens, tightens, and tones the entire upper abdominal area. Also helps to strengthen the lower abdominal area.

STANCE: Lie flat on your back on the floor, and pull your knees up until your legs form an L. You may cross your feet at the ankles. Place your hands behind your head.

MOVEMENT: Flexing your upper abdominal muscles as hard as possible, raise your shoulders off the floor in a curling movement until your shoulders are completely off the ground, all the time keeping your knees raised so that your legs form an L shape. Without resting, and keeping the pressure on your upper abdominal area, return to start position. Repeat this movement until you have completed your set. Rest zero to fifteen seconds, and do a second set of the bent-knee leg raise and the knee-raised crunch. (You will do three sets of this exercise combination in all and then proceed to the last abdominal exercise, the oblique crunch and, if you choose the option, the reverse crunch).

Remember, you will do three sets of fifteen to twenty-five repetitions for each abdominal exercise.

ALERT: This is exactly the same movement as the crunch, only it is done with the knees raised. Do not hold your breath. Breathe naturally.

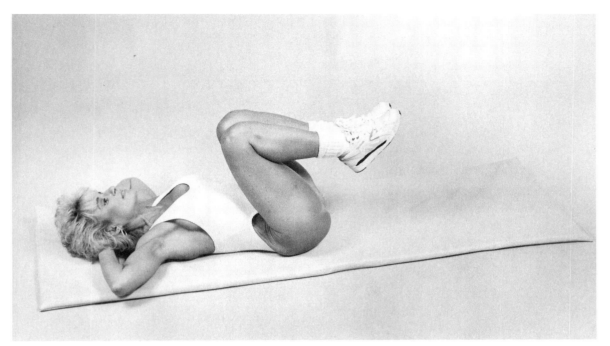

Start

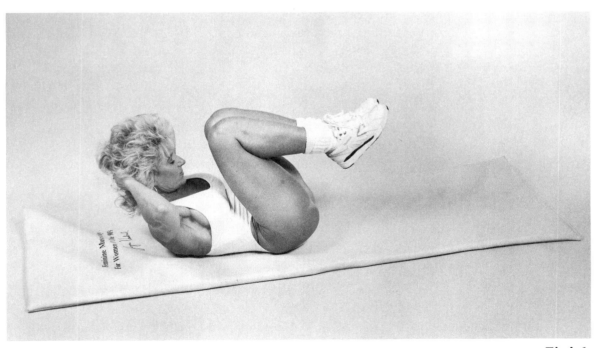

Finish

3. Oblique Crunch and (Optional) Reverse Crunch

Side Abdominals: Oblique Crunch

Develops, strengthens, and defines the side abdominal muscles (obliques) and strengthens the upper and lower abdominal muscles.

STANCE: Lie flat on your back on the floor, and bend your knees. Place your feet together and let your legs fall to one side until your lower knee is touching the floor. Place your hands behind your head.

MOVEMENT: Keeping your back as flat to the ground as possible, raise just your shoulders off the floor until you are in the crunch position. Be sure to move up in a straight line and to lift from the chest and not the neck. Keeping the pressure on your working oblique muscles, return to start position and repeat the movement until you have completed your set. Repeat the set for the other side of your body. If you are not doing the optional twin to this set, rest zero to fifteen seconds and perform a second and third set. Congratulations. You have completed your lower and middle body workouts for workout day one. If you are doing the optional twin for this set, the reverse crunch, proceed to that exercise without resting. (See page 120 for the reverse crunch.)

Remember that you always do fifteen to twenty-five repetitions in each set for all abdominal exercises.

ALERT: It will be tempting to allow your shoulders to move to one side or the other while you are performing this exercise. Try to keep your shoulders straight and your chest facing straight to the ceiling throughout the movement.

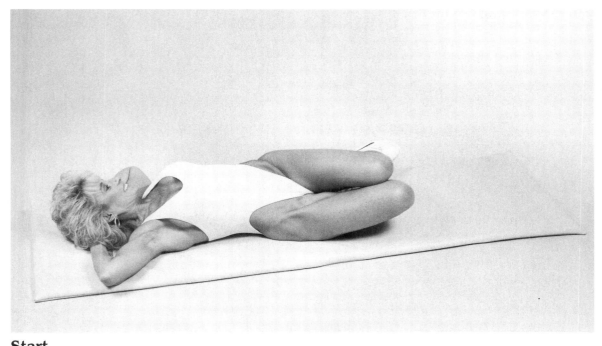

Start

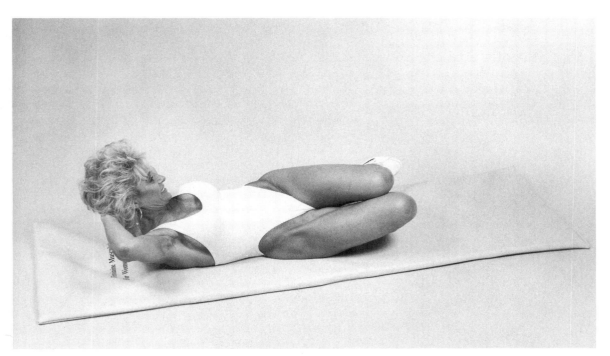

Finish

REVIEW OF EXERCISES IN THIS CHAPTER

THIGH—HIP/BUTTOCK INTERSETS

Thighs	Hips/Buttocks
1. Plié squat (*or* lying one-legged inner-thigh squeeze)	**1.** Standing back leg extension
2. Bugs Bunny lunge (*or* standing one-legged thigh sweep)	**2.** Standing butt squeeze
3. Sissy squat (*or* modified sissy squat)	**3.** Straight-leg kick-up
4. Leg extension	**4.** Vertical scissor
5. Hack squat (*or* toes-pointed-out leg extension)	**5.** Feather kick-up
6. Leg curl	**6.** Prone butt lift
7. Lying inner-thigh scissor	**7.** Lying butt lift

LOWER AND UPPER ABDOMINAL INTERSETS

Lower Abdominals

1. Knee-in (*or* reverse crunch)

2. Bent-knee leg raise (*or* six-inch leg raise)

Upper Abdominals

1. Crunch

2. Bent-knee sit-up (*or* knee-raised crunch)

Side Abdominals (Obliques)

3. Oblique crunch

3. Reverse crunch (*optional*)

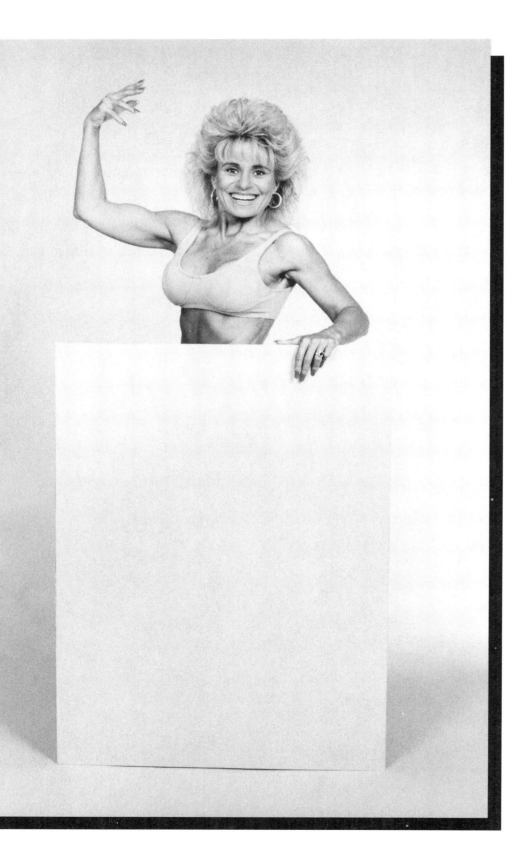

6

DAY TWO—
UPPER BODY
WORKOUT

Many women are not overly concerned with the development of the upper body and would even choose to skip over that area when working out, believing that they should save all of their energy for the places where they really need the work. While these women have a point—and indeed they are right to place special emphasis where it's needed (the lower and middle body)—to completely neglect the upper body would be a BIG MISTAKE.

To refuse to exercise the upper body would be to create an imbalanced body with firm, shapely hips and buttocks, a flat, well-defined stomach— and soft, flabby arms, drooping shoulders, a sagging chest, and a fatty back. Not only is such a body unappealing—indeed, not sexy—but it isn't healthy! It creates poor posture caused by muscular imbalance—and eventually back, neck, and shoulder problems.

Fortunately the upper body does not require as much work as the lower body. Although the upper body workout includes more body parts than the lower and middle body workout, there are less exercises required for each part. Whereas you performed seven exercises each for buttocks and thighs, and five exercises for abdominals, nineteen exercises in all, you will perform only three exercises for each of the six upper body parts—eighteen exercises in all. So don't worry that you're going to be "in for it" today. The workout is equally balanced.

Just the way you may have been surprised to find that you were no longer exhausted when you exercised your lower body and middle body, chances are you will feel the same way when you work on your upper body. You will again work in twin sets, doing one set for, say, the chest and then, while your chest muscles are resting, one set for the shoulders, and so on until your chest-shoulder routine is finished. When you are done, you will wonder why the routine seems to have gone so fast. Then of course you will remember that you are working in intersets, carefully paired exercises selected for energy efficiency and elimination of boredom.

THE UPPER BODY WORKOUT

You will be doing three twin sets of exercises for each pair: chest and shoulders, biceps and triceps, and back and calves. The body parts in the first two pairs are grouped together because they are closely related, and the muscles "tie in" with each other. The back-calf pair is an exception. This "odd couple" is matched because they both happen to be left without a partner. Although strange bedfellows, they do make a neat pair, because they are both relatively easy to exercise and they are placed at the very end of the workout—as a "carrot on the stick." If you get through the first two pairs and you feel a bit tired and think of quitting, you can tell yourself, "Oh, well. I only have to do the back and calves. That's easy. I might as well finish."

CHEST-SHOULDER INTERSETS

Chest

1. Flat dumbbell press

2. Incline dumbbell flye

3. Cross-bench pullover

4. Incline dumbbell press (WW)

5. Flat dumbbell flye (T)

Shoulders

1. Seated side lateral

2. Seated alternate dumbbell press

3. Standing alternate front lateral raise

4. Seated bent lateral (WW)

5. Pee-wee lateral (T)

BICEPS-TRICEPS INTERSETS

Biceps

1. Seated simultaneous curl
2. Standing alternate hammer curl
3. Seated concentration curl
4. Seated alternate curl (WW)
5. Incline simultaneous hammer curl (T)

Triceps

1. Close bench triceps press
2. Flat cross-face triceps extension
3. One-arm overhead triceps extension
4. One-arm triceps kickback (WW)
5. Incline cross-face triceps extension (T)

BACK-CALF INTERSETS

Back

1. Leaning one-arm dumbbell row
2. Upright row
3. Seated dumbbell back lateral
4. Double-arm reverse row (WW)
5. Bent-knee dead lift (T)

Calves

1. Seated straight-toe calf raise
2. Standing straight-toe calf raise
3. Seated angled-in-toe calf raise
4. Seated angled-out-toe calf raise (WW)
5. Standing angle-out-toe calf raise (T)

Note: "WW" stands for the Wild Woman Workout, and "T" stands for the Terminator Workout. These workouts will be discussed later in this chapter.

How to Do the Upper Body Workout: Review

You do your first interset, the flat dumbbell press and the seated side lateral, without resting between sets. Then rest zero to fifteen seconds. Again, without breaking up the "Siamese twins," do a second set of that duet. Again rest zero to fifteen seconds, and complete your final twin set of that exercise combination. Now rest zero to fifteen seconds and move to your first interset of the next exercise combination, the incline dumbbell flye and the seated alternate dumbbell press. Rest zero to fifteen seconds . . . and so on until you have completed your entire upper body workout. (Note that there are no special rests allowed when you move to the next two body parts. You simply proceed as usual. You will be reminded of this fact in the exercise instructions.) For a full review on how to do the Bottoms Up! Workout, read chapter 4.

Sets, Repetitions, and Weight

You will use the modified pyramid system and do three sets of varying repetitions for each exercise:

> **Set 1:** twelve repetitions, three pounds
> **Set 2:** ten repetitions, five pounds
> **Set 3:** six to eight repetitions, eight pounds

If the above weights are too heavy, you may substitute one-pound dumbbells, two-pound dumbbells, and three-pound dumbbells. If they are too light, you may substitute three-pound dumbbells, five-pound dumbbells, and ten-pound dumbbells.

Dumbbell weights refer to **each** dumbbell. In other words, in the above example you will be holding one three-pound dumbbell in each hand, one five-pound dumbbell in each hand, and one eight-pound dumbbell in each hand.

Heaviness of Weights Will Later Depend upon the Body Part You Are Exercising!

Eventually, the weight you use will depend upon the body part you are exercising. But for now, to keep things simple, I prefer that you use the same weights for all body parts unless you are a seasoned weight-trainer.

Later you will use lighter weights for certain body parts and heavier ones for others. For example, later you will discover that you can use heavier weights for your chest, biceps, back, and calves than for your shoulder and triceps. (Weight for the abdominal workout is optional and will be discussed later.)

What If You Cannot Pyramid Certain Exercises?

You may find that the suggested weights are fine for most exercises, but for some you cannot advance to the higher weight for second and third sets because the weights are too heavy. This usually happens when it comes to training the shoulders and triceps. In such a case, simply keep the same weight for all three sets until you are strong enough to pyramid the weights (you will gain significant strength in three weeks' time).

As mentioned in chapter 5, it's a good idea to purchase sets of dumbbells in each of the following weights: three pounds, five pounds, and eight pounds. If you cannot find them in your local sporting goods store, you may order them from me. (See page 283.)

Raising the Weights As You Get Stronger

After working out for about three weeks, you may find that the weights you are using feel a bit too light. In other words, if you find yourself flying through the workout without a challenge, it's time to raise your overall weights. For example, if you were using dumbbells of three pounds, five pounds, and eight pounds, it's time to advance to dumbbells of five pounds, eight pounds, and ten pounds.

After, say, another month, you may find that again, the weights have become too easy. Now you may want to raise the weights again—say, to eights, tens, and twelves. It's not a good idea to raise the weights more than two to five pounds at a time.

The Plateau

Since this is a very intense workout, you cannot go extremely high in weight even if you want to. The highest weights you should ever use with this workout are dumbbells of ten, fifteen, and twenty pounds, unless of course you modify the workout as described below, in order to build larger muscles.

Heavier Weights and Longer Rests to Build Larger Upper-Body Muscles

If you want to build a larger muscle, you must use heavier weights and rest longer between sets. It's a good idea to build larger muscles for both members of a twin set because the twin sets are related in balanced pairs. In other words, you wouldn't want a larger biceps and a tiny triceps muscle because it would throw your arm out of balance. You wouldn't want strong chest muscles and weak shoulder muscles because it would throw off your posture. If you want a larger back but not larger calves, it's simple: just isolate them and work as you would in a regular bodybuilding routine, using heavy weights and taking forty-five to sixty-second rests between sets.

Why am I telling you all of this when you have enough trouble just learning the regular Bottoms Up! Workout? I have learned from experience that many women advance quickly and branch out on their own and want to change things. I get so many letters about this that I feel that I must give you some options ahead of time.

I suggest that unless you are an old hand at working out, you follow the program exactly as written for six months. Then you can experiment all you please.

Wild Woman and Terminator Workouts

As you may have noticed, wild woman and terminator workouts are not provided for the lower and middle body workouts. The reason is simple. They are already included in the workout. In short, they are mandatory. I have already required that you do seven exercises for the thighs and hip/buttocks, and five exercises for the abdominals. In short, I felt that I could give you no choice. If I am going to be responsible for the reshaping of your body, I have to give you a workout that is sure-fire! And I know full well that I can't give you the option of doing less work for those troublesome areas. They must be "bombed."

Not so with the upper body. Going the extra mile here is truly an option—unless of course you happen to have a particularly troublesome upper-body part. Then you will choose to do the Wild Woman or Terminator Workout for that part.

Here's how it works. If you want to do one extra exercise for a given body part, add the fourth exercise for both body parts in that twin set so that you will be doing a complete "interset" for that body part and its companion body part. You will then be doing the Wild Woman Workout, a total of four exercises for that body part.

If you want to do still more work for a given body part, add the fifth exercise for that part and its twin. You will then be doing the Terminator Workout, a total of five exercises for that body part.

You may choose to make your life simple and do the Wild Woman or Terminator routine for your entire upper body by doing a fourth and/or fifth exercise for all upper body parts, or you can pick and choose to do extra work on only certain body parts. For example, you may want stronger, more muscular arms, but not a stronger, more muscular chest-shoulder or back-calf area. If you feel this way, you can do Wild Woman and/or Terminator routines for your arms (biceps-triceps routine) but leave your chest-shoulders and back-calves at the regular three exercises. On the other hand, you may want something else—say, a stronger chest-shoulder area, but without extra work on your arms, and so on.

If you add an exercise for a body part that is paired with another, be sure to do the companion exercise so that you will continue to use the interset system and so that you will keep your muscular development for that body area balanced. Let me explain.

If you want to do extra work for your chest, you should also do extra work for your shoulders, since these two body parts work together. Making one stronger than the other may throw your body out of balance. The same holds true for the biceps and triceps—muscles located on either side of the arm. Frankly, the back and calves have no relation at all, so if you want to add exercises just for back but not the calves, or vice-versa, go right ahead. But this of course would have you doing that body part without a partner. It's up to you. I prefer that you do everything in intersets, just for the sake of consistency.

How Much Extra Time Will Wild Woman and Terminator Take?

Adding the Wild Woman Workout to your entire upper body will only add seven minutes to your routine, and adding the Terminator will add another seven minutes to your routine. If your regular workout took twenty minutes, you will then finish in twenty-seven to thirty-four minutes. (As mentioned before, don't be alarmed if the workout takes you a lot longer in the beginning, especially if you are new at working with weights or have not worked out in a long time. Soon you will pick up the pace.)

What If You Are Doing the Regular Upper Body Workout, but Hate One of the Exercises?

Good news. If you are doing the regular upper body workout and can't stand one of your exercises, you should feel free to substitute a wild woman or terminator exercise for it. In other words, you can use these exercises as variations. You don't have to substitute the pair—just the exercise you don't like. For example, in your biceps-triceps routine, suppose you like the seated simultaneous curl for your biceps, but you hate the close bench triceps press. You can replace the close bench triceps press with either the one-arm overhead triceps extension or the one-arm triceps kickback, which are found in the Wild Woman and Terminator routines; but keep your original biceps exercise, the seated simultaneous curl. As long as you give your biceps a triceps partner for that exercise, all is well.

Variations

Whether you are doing the regular, the Wild Woman, or the Terminator routines, you can use the variations anytime you choose, for the sake of variety or because you like the variation better.

CHEST-SHOULDER ROUTINE

1. Flat Dumbbell Press and Seated Side Lateral

Chest: Flat Dumbbell Press

Develops, shapes, and defines the entire chest (pectoral) area.

STANCE: Lie on a flat exercise bench with a dumbbell held in each hand, palms facing upward. The outer edge of the dumbbells should be touching your upper chest area.

MOVEMENT: Flexing your chest muscles, extend your arms upward until your elbows are nearly locked. The dumbbells should be in line with your upper chest in this fully extended position. Return to start and feel the stretch in your chest. Repeat the movement until you have completed your set. Without resting, proceed to the other exercise in this twin set, the seated side lateral.

ALERT: Maintain control of the dumbbells as you extend and lower your arms. Remember to flex your chest muscles on the upward movement and to stretch them on the downward movement. Keep your mind riveted on your chest muscles throughout the exercise.

VARIATION: You may perform this exercise with a barbell.

GYM WORKOUT: You may perform this exercise on any bench press machine.

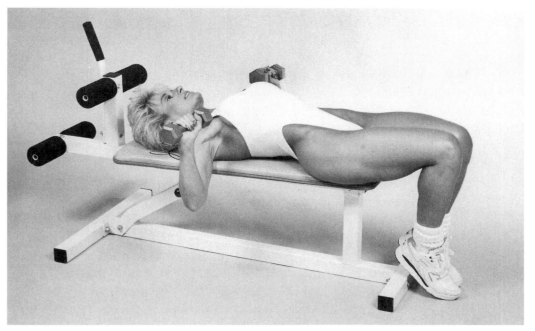

Start

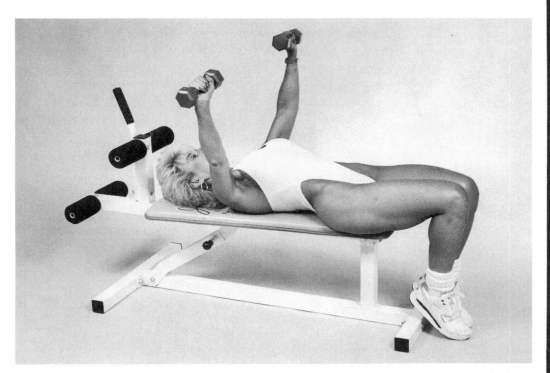

Finish

Shoulders: Seated Side Lateral

Develops and shapes the entire shoulder muscle (deltoid), especially the side (medial) area.

STANCE: Sit at the edge of a flat exercise bench with your feet together or a natural width apart. With a dumbbell in each hand, palms angled toward each other, hold the dumbbells centered in front of you, letting them touch at the edges. Sit up straight and keep your back erect.

MOVEMENT: Flexing your shoulder muscles as you go, extend your arms upward and outward until the dumbbells reach slightly higher than shoulder height. In full control, return to start position and repeat the movement until you have completed your set. Rest zero to fifteen seconds and do a second interset of the flat dumbbell press and the seated side lateral. (You will do three sets of this exercise combination in all and then proceed to the next exercise combination.)

Remember, you will do twelve repetitions for your first set of each chest and shoulder exercise, ten repetitions for your second set, and six to eight repetitions for your third set.

ALERT: Beware of the temptation to swing the dumbbells. Do not lean forward. Control the dumbbells. If the work is too hard, use lighter dumbbells. Don't hold your breath. Breathe naturally.

VARIATION: You may perform this exercise standing. It is a little easier to do that way because you are not isolating the muscle as completely.

GYM WORKOUT: You may perform this exercise on any side lateral machine.

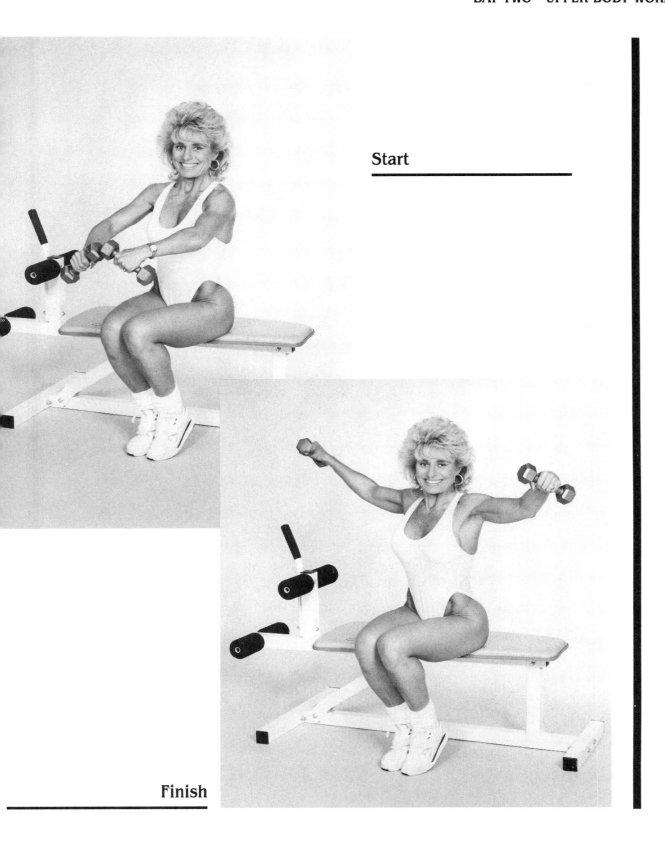

Start

Finish

2. Incline Dumbbell Flye and Seated Alternate Dumbbell Press

Chest: Incline Dumbbell Flye

Gives definition (cleavage) to the upper chest area and develops and shapes the entire chest (pectoral) area.

STANCE: Lie on an incline exercise bench with a dumbbell held in each hand, palms facing each other and elbows slightly bent. Extend your arms straight up and allow the dumbbells to touch each other. (Your extended arms and the dumbbells should be centered above your chest.)

MOVEMENT: Extend your arms outward and downward in an arclike movement until you feel a full stretch in your pectoral muscles. Flexing your chest muscles, return to start position and repeat the movement until you have completed your set. Without resting, proceed to the other exercise in this twin set, the seated alternate dumbbell press.

ALERT: Do not change the position of your arms as you work. Lock your elbows into a slightly bent position and leave them that way. Think of your arms as slightly curved steel bars that cannot be bent.

GYM WORKOUT: You may use the "peck deck" machine in place of this exercise.

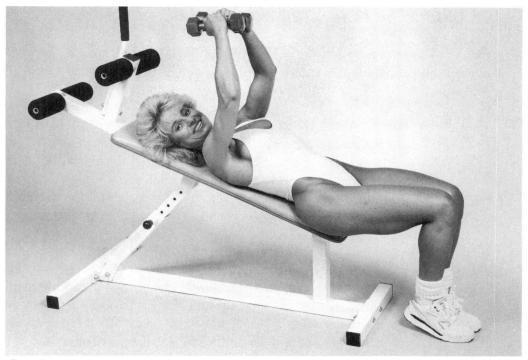

Start

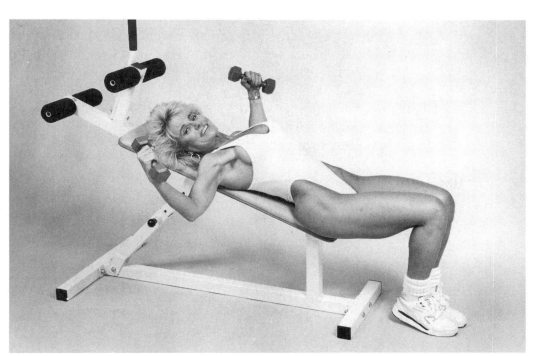

Finish

Shoulders: Seated Alternate Dumbbell Press

Develops and shapes the entire shoulder muscle (deltoid) and helps to give added definition to the front (anterior) shoulder muscle.

STANCE: Sit at the edge of a flat exercise bench, with your feet together or a natural width apart. Hold a dumbbell in each hand at shoulder height, palms facing away from your body. The ends of the dumbbells should graze your shoulders. Keep your back erect and look straight ahead.

MOVEMENT: Raise your right arm upward until it is fully extended. While returning your right arm to start position, raise your left arm upward until it is fully extended. Continue this alternating up-and-down movement until you have completed your set. Rest zero to fifteen seconds and do a second set of the incline dumbbell flye and the seated alternate dumbbell press. (You will do three sets of this exercise combination in all and then proceed to the next exercise combination.)

Remember, you will do twelve repetitions for your first set of each chest and shoulder exercise, ten repetitions for your second set, and six to eight repetitions for your last set.

ALERT: Do not allow your torso to rock from side to side. Do not lean forward or backward. Remember to flex your shoulders on each upward movement.

VARIATION: You may perform this exercise two arms at a time. You may perform this exercise standing. You may perform this exercise by placing a barbell behind your head and resting on your shoulders.

GYM WORKOUT: You may perform this exercise on any shoulder press machine.

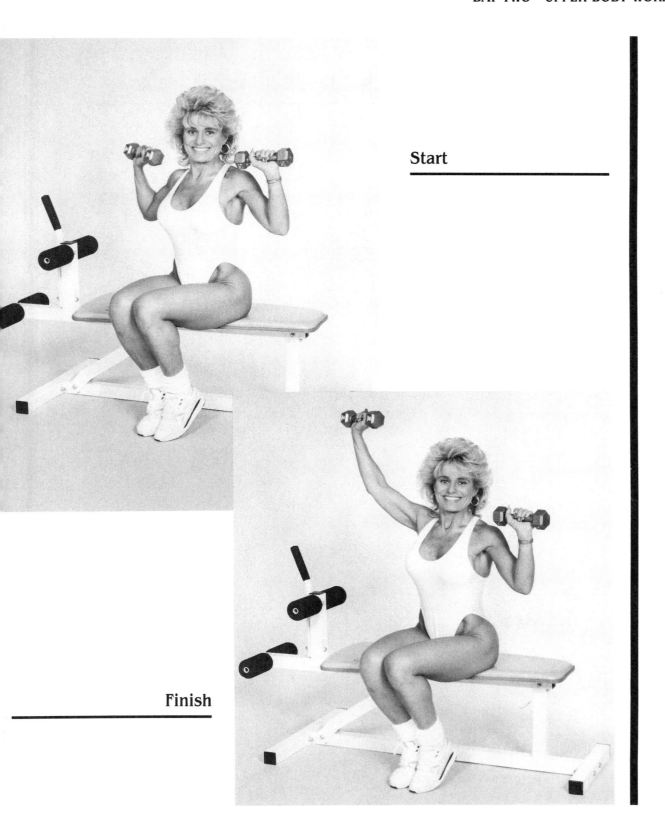

Start

Finish

3. Cross-Bench Pullover and Standing Alternate Front Lateral Raise

Chest: Cross-Bench Pullover

Develops and shapes the entire chest area. Also helps to expand the rib cage and stretch the back muscles (latissimus dorsi).

STANCE: Lie at the edge of a flat exercise bench with your shoulders touching the edge of the bench. Hold a dumbbell in your hands, palms upward, between your crossed thumbs. Extend your arms straight up so that the dumbbell is held directly over your forehead.

MOVEMENT: Lower the dumbbell behind you by lowering your arms and bending your elbows at the same time, until you cannot go any farther. Feel a full stretch in your pectoral muscles. Flex your chest muscles as you return to start position, and give your muscles an extra hard flex as you reach start position. Repeat the movement until you have completed your set. Without resting, proceed to the other exercise in this twin set, the standing alternate front lateral raise.

ALERT: Do not let the weight nearly fall to the down position. Maintain control at all times. Do not hold your breath. Breathe naturally.

VARIATION: You may perform this exercise in the traditional manner, with your feet on the ground and your shoulders resting on the edge of the bench. If you choose to use this method, remember to keep your buttocks down as you work.

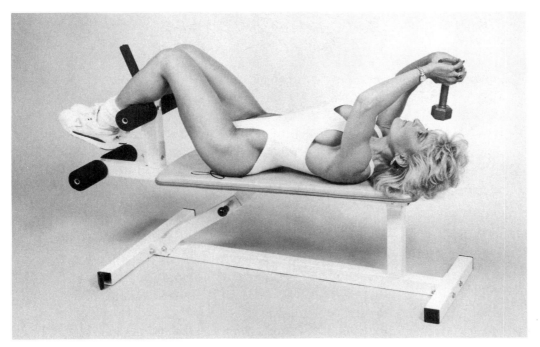

Start

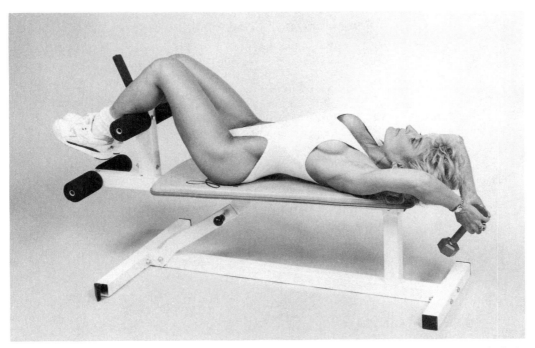

Finish

Shoulders: Standing Alternate Front Lateral Raise

Develops and shapes the front (anterior) shoulder muscle (deltoid).

STANCE: Stand with your feet a natural width apart. Hold a dumbbell in each hand, palms facing your body, and extend your arms straight down in front of you, so that the dumbbells are touching the center of your upper thighs.

MOVEMENT: Flexing your shoulder muscles, lock your elbows and extend one arm upward until it is parallel to the floor. As you begin to return to start position, start raising the other arm and do so until it is parallel to the floor. In the meantime, your other arm will have returned to start position. Continue to work in this manner until you have completed your set. Rest zero to fifteen seconds and do a second set of the cross-bench pullover and the standing alternate front lateral raise. (You will do three sets of this exercise combination in all and then proceed to the next muscle group, the biceps-triceps combination.)

Remember, do twelve repetitions for your first set of each chest and shoulder exercise, ten repetitions for your second set, and six to eight repetitions for your last set.

ALERT: Keep your arms close to the sides of your body at all times. Don't swing the dumbbells up or nearly let them drop down. Maintain full control.

VARIATION: You may perform this exercise two arms at a time. You may use a barbell instead of dumbbells.

Start

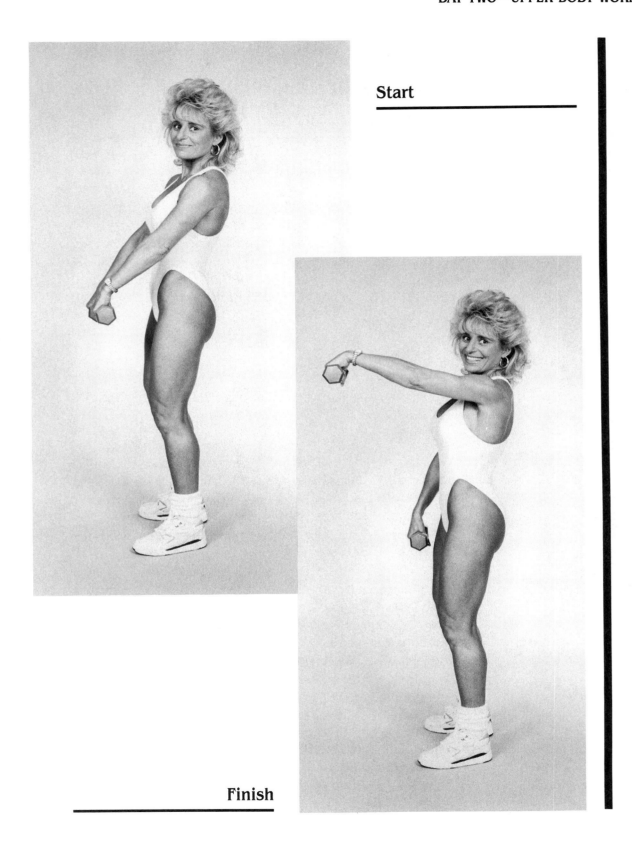

Finish

4. Incline Dumbbell Press and Seated Bent Lateral (for Wild Woman and Terminator Workouts)

Chest: Incline Dumbbell Press

Develops and tones the entire chest (pectoral) area, especially the upper chest area. Helps to give the look of cleavage to the breasts.

Perform this exercise exactly as you would the flat dumbbell press (see page 144), only use an incline exercise bench. You may adjust the incline to an approximate 30-degree angle. Do one set of this exercise, and without resting, proceed to the other exercise in this twin set, the seated bent lateral.

Shoulders: Seated Bent Lateral

Develops and shapes the rear (posterior) and side (medial) shoulder muscles (deltoids).

STANCE: Sit at the edge of a flat exercise bench, holding a dumbbell in each hand, palms facing each other. Bend over until your upper body is parallel to the floor (your chest should be resting upon your thigh muscles). Extend your arms straight down and touch the dumbbells together under your thighs.

MOVEMENT: Flexing your shoulder muscles and keeping your upper body down, extend your arms outward until they are nearly parallel to the floor (your elbows will be slightly bent in this position). Return to start and repeat the movement until you have completed your set. Rest zero to fifteen seconds and do another set of the incline dumbbell press and the seated bent lateral. (You will do three sets of this exercise combination in all and then proceed to the next exercise combination.)

Remember, you will do twelve repetitions for your first set of each chest and shoulder exercise, ten repetitions for your second set, and six to eight repetitions for your third set.

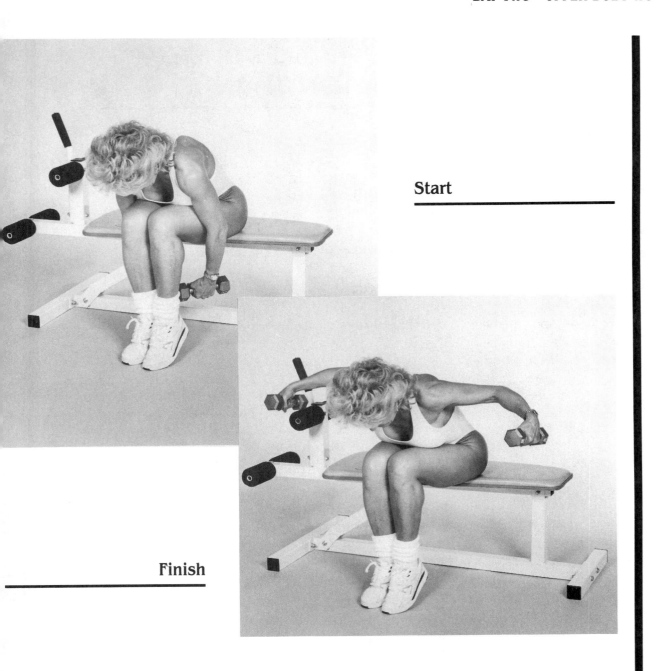

Start

Finish

ALERT: Beware of the temptation to rise up as you work. Keep your upper body in the torso-parallel-to-the-ground position throughout the movement.

VARIATION: You may perform this exercise standing.

5. Flat Dumbbell Flye and Pee-Wee Lateral (for Terminator Workout)

Chest: Flat Dumbbell Flye

Develops and shapes the entire chest (pectoral) area.

Perform this exercise in exactly the same manner as the incline dumbbell flye (see page 148), only use a flat exercise bench instead of an incline exercise bench. Perform one set of this exercise, and without resting, proceed to the other exercise in this twin set, the pee-wee lateral.

Shoulders: Pee-Wee Lateral

Develops, shapes, and defines the rear (posterior) and side (medial) shoulder muscles (deltoids).

STANCE: Stand with your feet together, and up on the toes of one foot. Hold a dumbbell in each hand, with your arms behind your back and your palms facing away from your body. The ends of the dumbbells should be touching each other. Bend at the knees and thrust your hips forward.

MOVEMENT: Flexing your shoulder muscles as you work, extend your arms outward and upward until the ends of the dumbbells reach ear height and are at arm's length on either side. Return to start position and repeat the movement until you have completed your set. Rest zero to fifteen seconds and do a second set of the flat dumbbell flye and the pee-wee lateral. (You will do three sets of this exercise combination in all and then proceed to the next exercise combination.)

Remember, you will do twelve repetitions for your first set of each chest and shoulder exercise, ten repetitions for your second set, and six to eight repetitions for your third set.

ALERT: Remember to flex and stretch your rear shoulder muscles as you raise and lower the dumbbells. Avoid rocking back and forth as you work. Move only your working arms. Don't hold your breath. Breathe naturally.

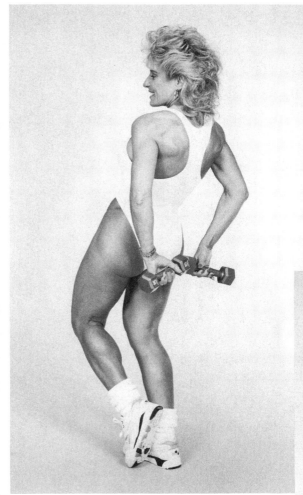

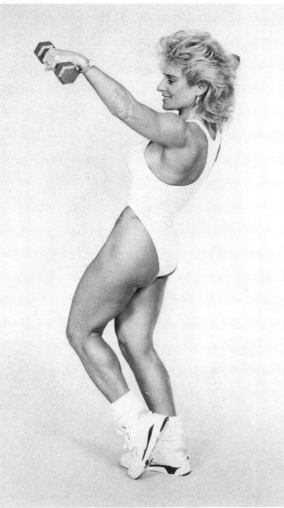

Start

Finish

BICEPS-TRICEPS ROUTINE

1. Seated Simultaneous Curl and Close Bench Triceps Press

Biceps: Seated Simultaneous Curl

Develops, shapes, and defines the entire biceps and helps to strengthen the forearm.

STANCE: Sit at the edge of a flat exercise bench, with your back erect and your feet together. Hold a dumbbell in each hand, palms facing forward. Place your arms straight down at your sides, and curl your wrists slightly upward. One end of each dumbbell should be touching your outer thigh.

MOVEMENT: Flexing your biceps as hard as possible and keeping your arms close to your body, curl your arms upward simultaneously until the dumbbells reach shoulder height and you cannot curl them any farther. In full control, return to start position and repeat the movement until you have completed your set. Without resting, proceed to the other exercise in this combination, the close bench triceps press.

ALERT: Do not lean forward or tip backward as you work. Don't jerk the dumbbells up or let them nearly drop to start position. Maintain control at all times.

VARIATION: You may perform this exercise standing, with dumbbells or with a barbell.

GYM WORKOUT: You may perform this exercise on any biceps curl machine.

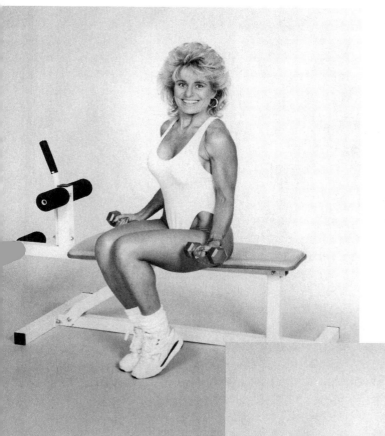

Start

Finish

Triceps: Close Bench Triceps Press

Develops, shapes, and defines the entire triceps.

STANCE: Lie on a flat exercise bench and grip a dumbbell in both hands, palms facing upward. Hold the dumbbell close to the center of your chest, and grip the ball at the end of the dumbbell with each hand.

MOVEMENT: Flexing your triceps as hard as possible, raise your arms upward until they are fully extended. Keeping your arms close to your body, return to start position and repeat the movement until you have completed your set. Rest zero to fifteen seconds and do a second set of the seated simultaneous curl and the close bench triceps press. (You will do three sets of this exercise combination in all, and then proceed to the next exercise combination.)

Remember, you will do twelve repetitions for your first set of each biceps and triceps exercise, ten repetitions for your second set, and six to eight repetitions for your third set.

ALERT: Keep your elbows close to your body as you raise and lower the dumbbell. This position ensures that your triceps are doing the work.

VARIATION: You may perform this exercise with a barbell.

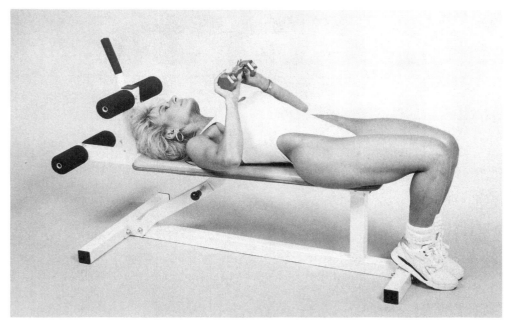

Start

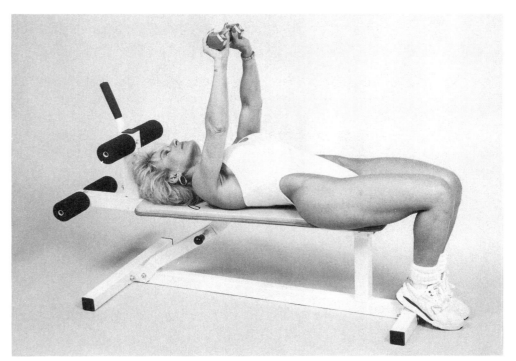

Finish

2. Standing Alternate Hammer Curl and Flat Cross-Face Triceps Extension

Biceps: Standing Alternate Hammer Curl

Develops and shapes the entire biceps. In addition, strengthens the forearm.

STANCE: Stand with your feet together. Hold a dumbbell in each hand, palms facing your body, and let your arms hang down at the sides of your body.

MOVEMENT: With palms facing your body and the dumbbells in the "hammer" position (see photograph), curl your right arm up to your right shoulder as far as you can. Begin to uncurl your right arm, at the same time curling your left arm up toward your left shoulder. Continue this alternating curl movement until you have completed your set. Without resting, proceed to the other exercise in this twin set, the flat cross-face triceps extension.

ALERT: Remember to flex your biceps on the upward movement and to feel the stretch on the downward movement. Beware of the temptation to rock your body back and forth in an effort to gain momentum and make the work easier. Remember: the more work you do, the better the results.

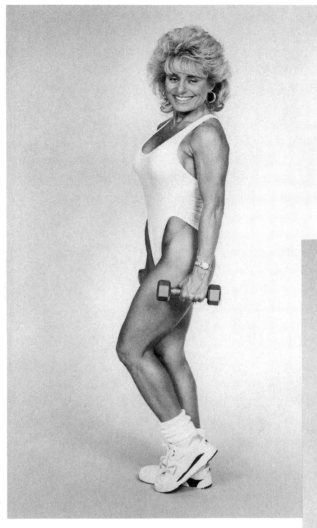

Start

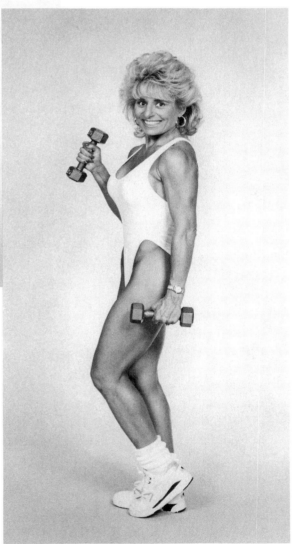

Finish

Triceps: Flat Cross-Face Triceps Extension

Develops and shapes the inner head of the triceps.

STANCE: Lie on a flat exercise bench with a dumbbell held straight up in your fully extended right arm, with your palm facing your legs. To avoid hitting yourself, turn your face so that your nose and mouth are touching your upper-arm area.

MOVEMENT: Bending your right arm at the elbow, lower your arm until the dumbbell touches your left neck-shoulder area. Flexing your triceps as hard as possible, return to start position and repeat the movement until you have completed your set. Repeat the set for the other arm. Rest zero to fifteen seconds and do a second set of the standing alternate hammer curl and the flat cross-face triceps extension. (You will do three sets of this exercise combination in all and then proceed to the next exercise combination.)

Remember, you will do twelve repetitions for your first set of each biceps-triceps combination, ten repetitions for your second set, and six to eight repetitions for your third set.

ALERT: Keep your mind riveted on your triceps as you work. Keep your working upper arm close to your body throughout the movement.

GYM WORKOUT: You may substitute for this exercise the triceps pushdown, which can be performed on any pulley with a triceps bar.

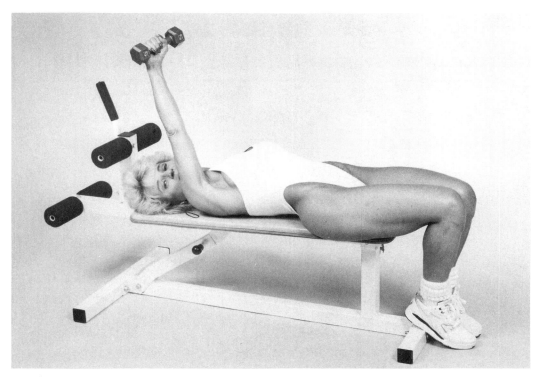

Start

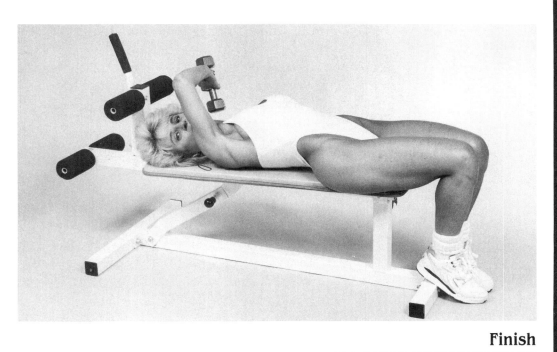

Finish

3. Seated Concentration Curl and One-Arm Overhead Triceps Extension

Biceps: Seated Concentration Curl

Develops, shapes, and defines the peak of the biceps. Also strengthens the forearm.

STANCE: Sit at the edge of a flat exercise bench and lean forward, placing your right elbow against your right inner knee. Hold a dumbbell in your right hand, palm away from your body. Extend your arm straight down. Keep your upper body down throughout the exercise.

MOVEMENT: Flexing your biceps as hard as possible, curl your right arm upward until the dumbbell reaches approximate chin height. Without looking up, return to start position and repeat the movement until you have completed your set. Perform the set for your other arm. Without resting, proceed to the other exercise in this twin set, the one-arm overhead triceps extension.

ALERT: Keep your elbow against your inner knee at all times. Do not fall into the trap of swinging the dumbbell to the up position and letting it nearly drop to the down position. Maintain control at all times.

VARIATION: You may perform this exercise in the traditional manner, while standing and leaning forward.

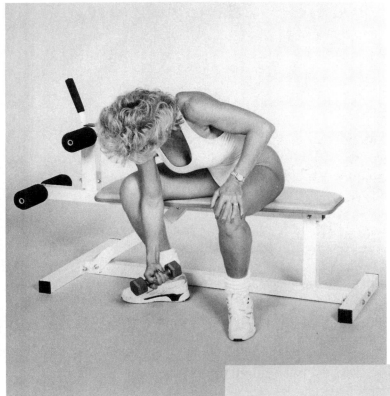

Start

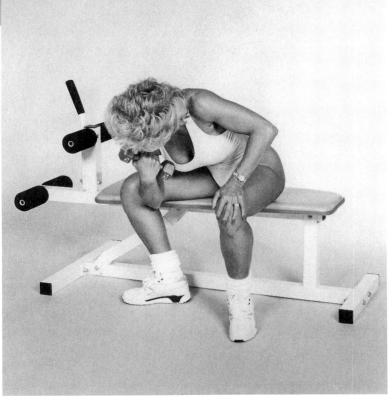

Finish

Triceps: One-Arm Overhead Triceps Extension

Develops, shapes, and defines the entire triceps, especially the inner and medial heads of that muscle.

STANCE: Stand with your feet in a comfortable position. Hold a dumbbell in your left hand, palm facing in toward your body, arm extended straight up, with your upper arm touching your ear.

MOVEMENT: Lower the dumbbell behind your head until it grazes your neck and upper back. Flexing your triceps as hard as possible, return to start position and repeat the movement until you have completed your set. Repeat the set for your right arm. Rest zero to fifteen seconds and do a second set of the seated combination curl and the one-arm overhead triceps extension. (You will do three sets of this exercise combination in all before beginning your first exercise combination for back and calves.)

Remember, you will do twelve repetitions for your first set of each biceps and triceps exercise, ten repetitions for your second set, and six to eight repetitions for your third set.

ALERT: Keep your upper arm close to your head at all times. You may place your nonworking fingertips on your working triceps so that you can feel your muscle expanding and contracting.

VARIATION: You may perform this exercise using two arms at a time and a heavier dumbbell.

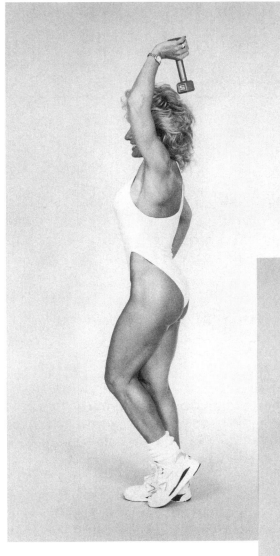

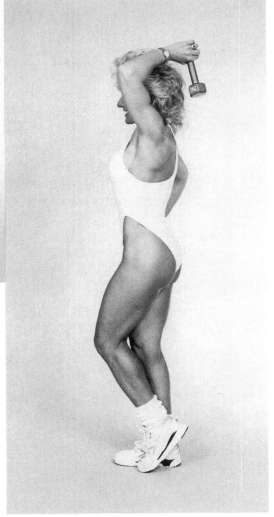

Start

Finish

4. Seated Alternate Curl and One-Arm Triceps Extension (for Wild Woman and Terminator Workouts)

Biceps: Seated Alternate Curl

Develops and shapes the entire biceps. In addition, strengthens the forearm.

You will perform this exercise in exactly the same manner as the seated simultaneous curl (see page 160), only you will alternate arms instead of curling both arms at a time. After you have performed a set of this exercise, without resting, proceed to the other exercise in this twin set, the one-arm triceps kickback.

Triceps: One-Arm Triceps Kickback

Develops and shapes the entire triceps.

STANCE: Stand with your feet together, bending at the waist and at the knees, and hold a dumbbell in your left hand, palm facing your body. Bend your left arm at the elbow so that your left forearm is nearly parallel to the floor and your elbow is touching your waist.

MOVEMENT: Keeping your upper arm close to your body, and flexing your triceps as you go, extend your left arm back as far as possible. Without resting, return to start position and repeat the movement until you have completed your set. Repeat the set for your right arm. Rest zero to fifteen seconds and do a second set of seated alternate curl and the one-arm triceps kickback. (You will do three sets of this exercise combination in all and then proceed to next exercise combination.)

Remember, you will do twelve repetitions for your first set of each biceps and triceps exercise, ten repetitions for your second set, and six to eight repetitions for your third set.

ALERT: Keep your upper arm as close to your body as possible as you work. Don't hold your breath. Breathe naturally.

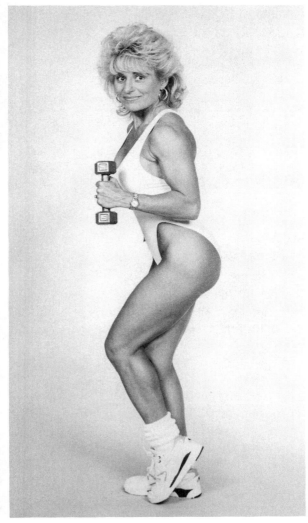

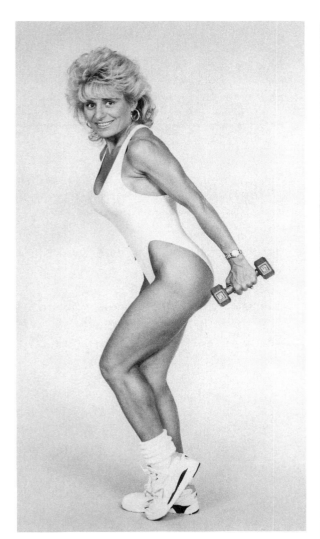

Start

Finish

VARIATION: You may perform this exercise by leaning with one knee on a flat exercise bench. You may do this exercise two arms at a time.

GYM WORKOUT: You may perform this exercise with a pully on any gym floor pulley device.

5. Incline Simultaneous Hammer Curl and Incline Cross-Face Triceps Extension (for Terminator Workout)

Biceps: Incline Simultaneous Hammer Curl

Strengthens, develops, and shapes the entire biceps.

Perform this exercise in exactly the same manner as the standing alternate hammer curl (see page 164), only lie on an incline bench and hammer with both arms at once instead of alternating arms.

After you have performed one set of this exercise, proceed without resting to the other exercise in this twin set, the incline cross-face triceps extension.

Triceps: Incline Cross-Face Triceps Extension

Strengthens, tones, and defines the entire triceps, especially the outer head of that muscle.

Perform this exercise in exactly the same manner as the flat cross-face triceps extension (see page 166), only lie on an incline bench.

After you have performed one set of this exercise, rest zero to fifteen seconds and do a second set of the incline simultaneous hammer curl and the incline cross-face triceps extension. (You will do three sets of this exercise combination in all and then proceed to the first interset in the back-calf routine.)

Remember, you will do twelve repetitions for your first set of each biceps and triceps exercise, ten repetitions for your second set, and six to eight repetitions for your third set.

BACK-CALF ROUTINE

1. Leaning One-Arm Dumbbell Row and Seated Straight-Toe Calf Raise

Back: Leaning One-Arm Dumbbell Row

Develops, strengthens, shapes, and defines the back muscles (latissimus dorsi) and helps to develop the biceps.

STANCE: Bend at the waist, with a dumbbell held in your left hand, palm facing your body. Place your right hand in a comfortable position, out of the way. Extend your left arm straight down until you feel the stretch in your latissimus dorsi muscle.

MOVEMENT: Raise your left arm to waist level while at the same time flexing your back muscles to the fullest extent. Continue to raise the dumbbell until your elbow is extended beyond your waist. Without resting, and keeping your arm as close to your body as possible, return to start position and repeat the movement until you have completed your set. Perform the set for the other side of your body. Without resting, proceed to the other exercise in this twin set, the seated straight-toe calf raise.

ALERT: Remember to maintain full control of the dumbbell. Do not hold your breath. Breathe naturally.

VARIATION: You may perform this exercise two arms at a time.

GYM WORKOUT: You may substitute this exercise for the lat pulldown to the front or back.

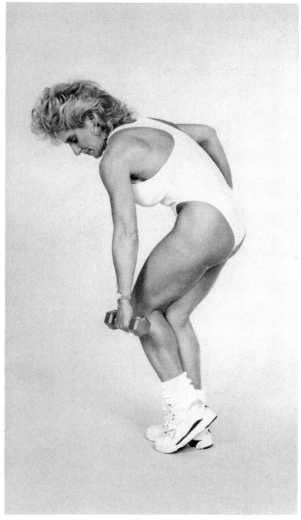

Finish

Start

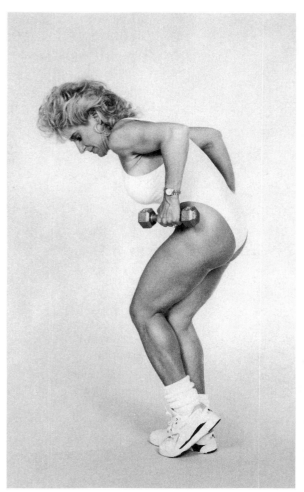

Calves: Seated Straight-Toe Calf Raise

Develops and shapes the entire calf muscle (gastrocnemius).

STANCE: Sit on the edge of a flat exercise bench, with a set of dumbbells held on the top of your knees. Plant your heels on the ground.

MOVEMENT: Keeping your toes pointed straight ahead and flexing your calf muscles as hard as possible, raise your heels until you cannot go any farther. Without resting, return to start position and repeat the movement until you have completed your set. Rest zero to fifteen seconds and do a second set of the leaning one-arm dumbbell row and the seated straight-toe calf raise. (You will do three sets of this exercise combination in all and then proceed to the next exercise combination.)

Remember, you will do twelve repetitions for your first set of each back and calf exercise, ten repetitions for your second set, and six to eight repetitions for your third set.

VARIATION: You may place the soles of your feet on a thick book for further stretch and flex of the calf muscles.

GYM WORKOUT: You may perform this exercise on any seated calf machine.

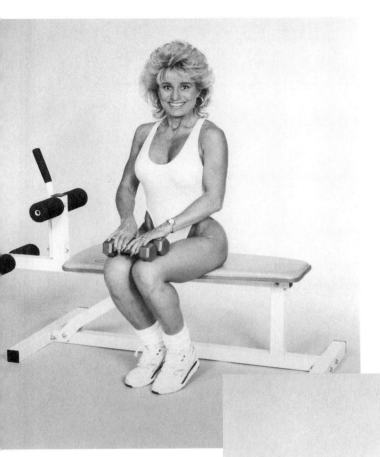

Start

Finish

2. Upright Row and Standing Straight-Toe Calf Raise

Back: Upright Row

Develops, shapes, and defines the entire trapezius muscle. It also strengthens the front (anterior) shoulder muscle (deltoid).

STANCE: Stand with your feet a natural width apart, and hold a dumbbell with both hands in the center of the dumbbell, palms facing your body. Extend your arms fully downward, and keep the dumbbell close to your body and centered.

MOVEMENT: Flexing your shoulder and trapezius muscles as hard as possible, extending your elbows outward, and keeping the dumbbell close to your body, raise the dumbbell until it reaches chin height. Flex your shoulder and trapezius an extra pinch and return to start position. Repeat the movement until you have completed your set. Without resting, proceed to the other exercise in this twin set, the standing straight-toe calf raise.

ALERT: Keep the dumbbell close to your body throughout the exercise. Do not shorten the movements. Be sure to go all the way up to chin level on each up movement and to descend all the way down until your arms are fully stretched on the down movement.

VARIATION: You may use a barbell to perform this exercise.

GYM WORKOUT: You may perform this exercise by attaching a bar to any gym floor-pulley machine.

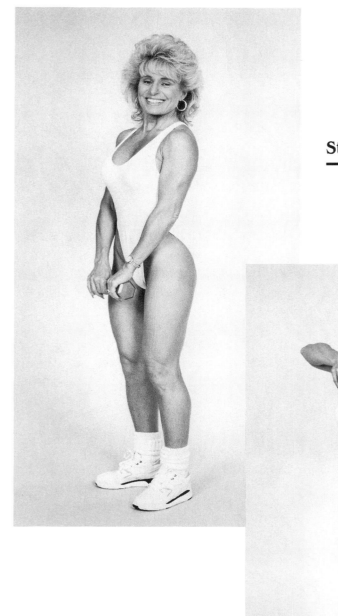

Start

Finish

Calves: Standing Straight-Toe Calf Raise

Develops, defines, and shapes the entire calf muscle (gastrocnemius).

STANCE: Stand with your feet a natural width apart, and your feet flat on the floor.

MOVEMENT: Flexing your left calf muscle, raise yourself onto your toes as high as possible. When you reach the highest point, give your calf muscle an extra-hard flex. Return to start position and repeat the movement until you have completed your set. Repeat the movement for the right calf. Rest zero to fifteen seconds and do a second set of the upright row and the standing straight-toe calf raise. (You will do three sets of this exercise combination in all, then proceed to the next exercise combination.)

Remember, you will do twelve repetitions for your first set of each back and calf exercise, ten repetitions for your second set, and six to eight repetitions for your third set.

ALERT: You may be tempted to descend to less than lowest level, or to ascend to less than highest level in an effort to cut the movement short and make the work easier. Don't do it. Perform full repetitions each time.

VARIATION: You may perform this exercise on the edge of a stair. You may perform this exercise by placing the sole of your working calf on the edge of a thick book, in order to get a fuller stretch and flex in the calf muscle.

GYM WORKOUT: You may perform this exercise on any standing calf machine.

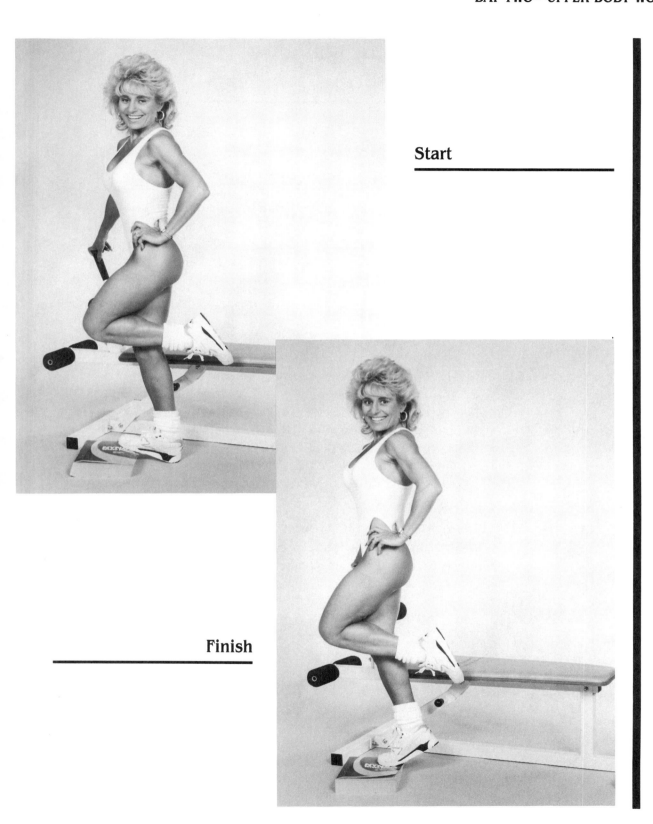

Start

Finish

3. Seated Dumbbell Back Lateral and Seated Angled-In-Toe Calf Raise

Back: *Seated Dumbbell Back Lateral*

Develops, shapes, and defines the upper back and trapezius muscles.

STANCE: Holding a dumbbell in each hand, sit at the edge of a flat exercise bench and lean forward until your upper body is nearly parallel to the floor. Palms facing to the rear, hold the dumbbells behind your calves. Let the dumbbells touch each other.

MOVEMENT: Flexing your back muscles as hard as possible and keeping the dumbbells close to your legs at all times, raise the dumbbells up and back. Rotate the dumbbells 90 degrees as you go along, so that when you reach hip level, your palms are angled to the front and one end of each dumbbell is touching your hip area. Make believe you are trying to squeeze a pencil in the middle of your back on the up movement. Return to start position and feel a full stretch. Repeat the movement until you have completed your set. Without resting, proceed to the other exercise in this twin set, the seated angled-in-toe calf raise.

ALERT: Control the dumbbells at all times. Do not let them nearly drop to the start position. Keep your arms as close to your sides as you work.

GYM WORKOUT: You may substitute any T-bar rowing machine.

Calves: *Seated Angled-In-Toe Calf Raise*

Develops, strengthens, and defines the outer calf area.

You will perform this exercise exactly the way you perform the seated straight-toe calf raise (see page 178), only you will angle your toes inward as far as possible.

After you have performed one set of this exercise, rest zero to fifteen seconds and do a second set of the seated dumbbell back lateral and the seated angled-in-toe calf raise. (You will do three sets of this exercise combination in all.)

Congratulations. You have completed your upper body workout. With this workout and yesterday's, you have exercised your entire body.

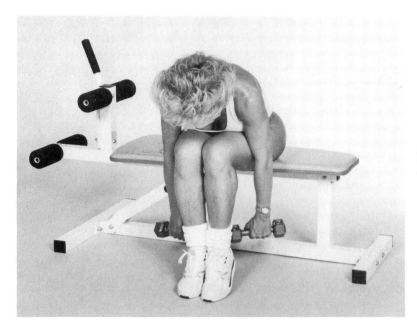

Start

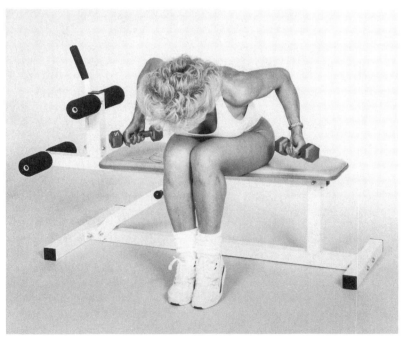

Finish

4. Double-Arm Reverse Row and Seated Angled-Out-Toe Calf Raise (for Wild Woman and Terminator Workouts)

Back: Double-Arm Reverse Row

Develops, defines, and shapes the latissimus dorsi, the trapezius, the rear deltoid, and the forearm.

STANCE: Stand with your feet shoulder-width apart, with a dumbbell held in each hand, palms away from your body. Bend over until your torso is parallel to the floor. Extend your arms straight down and keep them six inches away from the sides of your legs.

MOVEMENT: Raise the dumbbells up until they reach waist height, while at the same time flexing your latissimus dorsi muscles. Lower the dumbbells to start position and feel a full stretch in your back muscles. Repeat the movement until you have completed your set. Without resting, proceed to the other exercise in this twin set, the seated angled-out-toe calf raise.

ALERT: Maintain full control of the dumbbells at all times. Do not jerk them up or nearly let them drop to start position. Keep your back parallel to the floor throughout the exercise.

VARIATION: You may perform this exercise with a barbell.

GYM WORKOUT: For this exercise you may substitute the pulley row, done on any pulley rowing machine.

Calves: Seated Angled-Out-Toe Calf Raise

Develops, strengthens, and defines the inner calf muscle (gastrocnemius).

Perform this exercise in exactly the same manner as the seated-toe calf raise (see page 178), but instead of pointing your toes straight ahead, angle them out as far as possible and keep them angled out throughout the exercise. After you have performed your set for this exercise, rest zero to fifteen seconds and then do a second set of the double-arm reverse row and the seated angled-out-toe calf raise. (You will do three sets of this exercise combination in all. If you wish to do the Terminator Workout, you will then proceed to the next exercise combination.)

Remember, do twelve repetitions for your first set of each back and calf exercise, ten repetitions for your second set, and six to eight repetitions for your third set.

Start

Finish

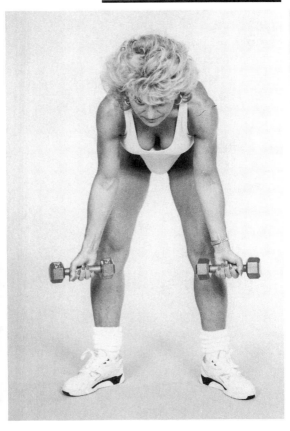
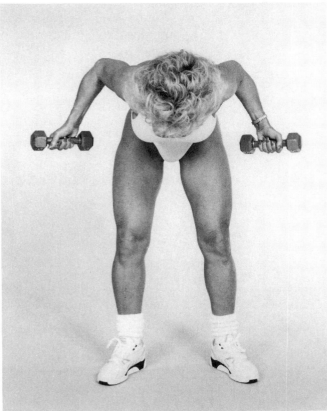

5. Bent-Knee Dead Lift and Standing Angled-Out-Toe Calf Raise

Back: Bent-Knee Dead Lift

Develops, shapes, and tones the back muscles (latissimus dorsi and trapezius).

STANCE: Place dumbbells on the floor in front of you, a little farther apart than shoulder width. With your feet a natural width apart, bend at the knees and grip the dumbbells, palms facing your body.

MOVEMENT: Flexing your back muscles as you move, rise to a standing position while at the same time keeping your eyes straight ahead. Without resting, raise your shoulders up and back as if you were shrugging your shoulders. With your arms straight down and your back straight, return to start position and repeat the movement until you have completed your set. Without resting, proceed to the other exercise in this twin set, the standing angled-out-toe calf raise.

ALERT: Do not hold your breath. Breathe naturally.

VARIATION: You may perform this exercise with a barbell.

Start

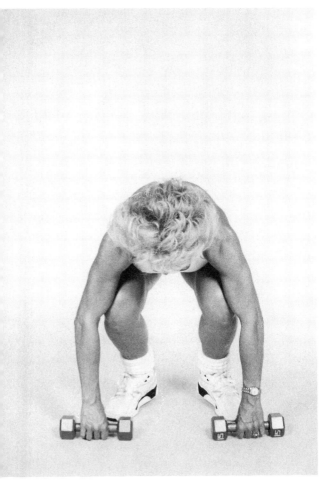

Finish

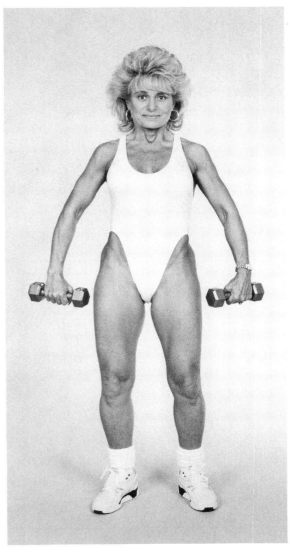

Calves: Standing Angled-Out-Toe Calf Raise

Develops, shapes, and defines the inner calf (gastrocnemius) area.

You will perform this exercise in exactly the same manner as the standing straight-toe calf raise (see page 182), only instead of pointing your toes straight ahead, you will angle them out to the side as far as possible. After you do one set of this exercise, rest for zero to fifteen seconds and do a second set of the bent-knee dead lift and the standing angled-out-toe calf raise. (You will do three sets of this exercise combination in all.)

Remember, you will do twelve repetitions for your first set of each back and calf exercise, ten repetitions for your second set, and six to eight repetitions for your last set.

REVIEW OF EXERCISES IN THIS CHAPTER

CHEST-SHOULDER INTERSETS

Chest

1. Flat dumbbell press
2. Incline dumbbell flye
3. Cross-bench pullover

4. Incline dumbbell press (WW)
5. Flat dumbbell flye (T)

Shoulders

1. Seated side lateral
2. Seated alternate dumbbell press
3. Standing alternate front lateral raise

4. Seated bent lateral (WW)
5. Pee-wee lateral (T)

BICEPS-TRICEPS INTERSETS

Biceps	**Triceps**
1. Seated simultaneous curl	1. Close bench triceps press
2. Standing alternate hammer curl	2. Flat cross-face triceps extension
3. Seated concentration curl	3. One-arm overhead triceps extension
4. Seated alternate curl (WW)	4. One-arm triceps kickback (WW)
5. Incline simultaneous hammer curl (T)	5. Incline cross-face triceps extension (T)

BACK-CALF INTERSETS

Back

1. Leaning one-arm dumbbell row

2. Upright row

3. Seated dumbbell back lateral

4. Double-arm reverse row (WW)

5. Bent-knee dead lift (T)

Calves

1. Seated straight-toe calf raise

2. Standing straight-toe calf raise

3. Seated angled-in-toe calf raise

4. Seated angled-out-toe calf raise (WW)

5. Standing angled-out-toe calf raise (T)

Note: "WW" stand for the "wild woman" workout, and "T" stands for the "terminator" workout.

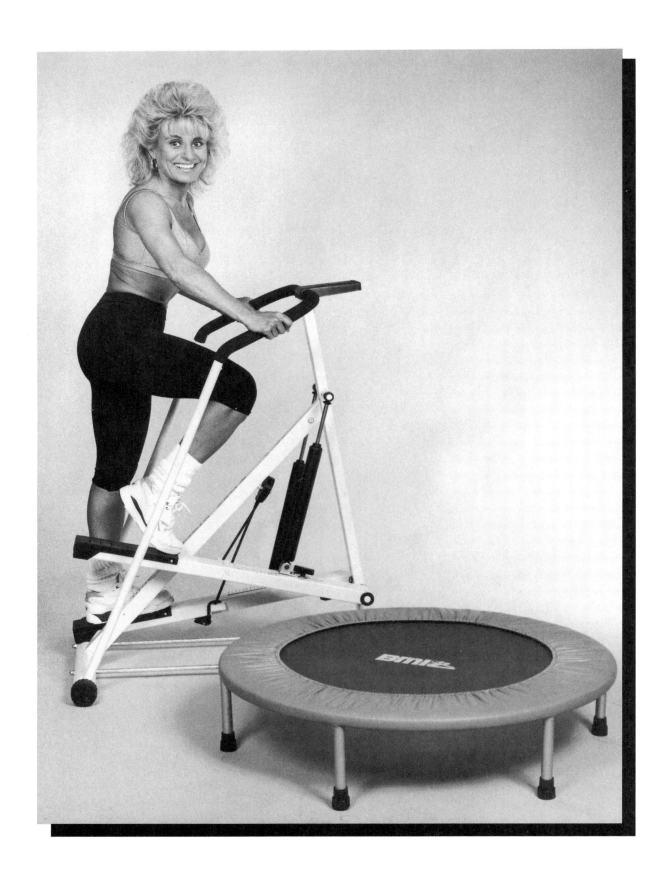

7
AEROBICS

Since the Bottoms Up! Workout is in and of itself an aerobic activity (it keeps your heart rate between 60 and 70 percent of capacity for twenty minutes or more), why is it a good idea to perform additional aerobic activities? How much fat can you burn in a given amount of time by performing specific aerobic activities? Is it possible to get a "semi-aerobic" fat-burning effect by engaging in lighter activities such as housecleaning or gardening? What about sports? Is it a waste of time to perform an aerobic or semi-aerobic activity for less than twenty minutes? These and other important questions will be discussed in this chapter, before I help you to create your workout schedule in chapter 8.

HOW AND WHY BOTTOMS UP! IS AN AEROBIC ACTIVITY

For an exercise to be officially considered aerobic, there are two requirements:

195

1. It must involve the movement of the large muscles of the body in a continual rhythmic manner for twenty minutes or more.
2. It must keep the pulse rate up between 60 and 85 percent of capacity. (Note that the lower end of the scale has been modified downward from 70 percent. It has now been discovered that the fat-burning aerobic effect is attained ideally in the 60 to 70 percent range.)

If Bottoms Up! is a weight-training routine, how can it be considered an aerobic activity? Isn't it true that weight training has traditionally been categorized as an "anaerobic" activity, and isn't it in fact the opposite of aerobic. (The word *aerobic* literally means with oxygen. As you perform an aerobic activity, the amount of oxygen your muscles need is continuously supplied. You are not forced to stop for a breath. *Anaerobic* literally means without oxygen. Your working muscles require more oxygen than your circulatory system can produce, so you are forced to stop for a breath.)

The answer to the seeming enigma lies in one simple fact. The kind of weight training that is considered to be anaerobic is heavy-weight training, where the individual must stop and take a significant rest between each set in order to regain enough oxygen and muscle recuperation to continue working out. In the Bottoms Up! Workout you will be working with light enough weights so that once you have become accustomed to the program and have passed your breaking-in period, you will rarely have to stop for a breath. (By the way, even if you take advantage of the optional short rest intervals, you will still have 90 percent of the aerobic effect and will burn about 90 percent of the fat you would burn if you didn't rest at all.)

WHY IS IT A GOOD IDEA TO INCLUDE "REGULAR" AEROBIC ACTIVITIES IN ADDITION TO BOTTOMS UP! IN YOUR FITNESS PLAN?

If you are too busy to include both aerobics and weight training, but you want to have the benefits of both, workouts such as this one and the Fat-Burning Workout are ideal. They accomplish muscle shaping and strengthening, bone strengthening, and fat burning, and they increase the heart and lung capacity. And you get all of this in one activity—working with light weights and taking few rests or none.

If you have time for additional exercise activity, however, you should choose to do additional aerobic activities as a first choice, and sports that give a semi-aerobic effect as a second choice. Why?

Regular aerobic activities are the best way to burn additional fat and to strengthen heart and lung capacity. Also, the fact is the Bottoms Up! Workout allows periodic fifteen-second rests (if you choose to take them). Straight aerobic activities such as running, stair stepping, or aerobic dance—in which no rests are taken whatsoever—ensure a full challenge to your heart and lungs. In addition, there is a carryover effect from aerobics into your Bottoms Up! Workout so that you will be able to perform Bottoms Up! with even more energy—and you may eventually be able to eliminate the rests completely. (Incidentally, you will note that the Bottoms Up! Workout also helps to increase your capacity in your aerobic activity. In other words, there is a mutual benefit.)

HOW CAN YOU TELL IF YOU ARE IN THE "AEROBIC RANGE" OF FAT-BURNING CAPACITY?

In order to determine your minimum and maximum aerobic pulse rate, subtract your age from 220. Then multiply the result by 60 percent. This will give you the minimum rate for the fat-burning aerobic range. Now multiply the figure by 70 percent. This will give you the maximum range for the ideal fat-burning aerobic effect. If you want to find your highest allowed aerobic range, after subtracting your age from 220, multiply the result by 85 percent. This is an excellent rate for increasing heart and lung capacity (you should of course build up to that range gradually), but it is *not* the ideal range for fat-burning. You will know that you are close to the 85 percent range when you are unable to speak to someone while performing the activity without gasping for air.

This brings me to my next point. I know that most health and fitness centers encourage stopping every so often and checking the pulse rate to see if one is in one's desired aerobic range. If you are like me and do not wish to interrupt your workout to do such checking, here is a simple rule of thumb. You will know that you are in the ideal fat-burning aerobic range of 60 to 70 percent of capacity if you feel you are working hard and

198

you break a sweat after about five to seven minutes—but can still, at any point during your activity, answer a civil question without gasping for breath. The bottom line is this: to burn maximum fat—good news!—you don't have to kill yourself, and you don't have to continually monitor yourself (unless of course your doctor advises that you do so). You simply have to "keep it moving" at a steady pace and feel as if you are working hard. (If you are curious, there's no reason why you can't check your pulse once you have finished your aerobic activity.)

HOW MUCH FAT DO VARIOUS AEROBIC ACTIVITIES BURN?

Some aerobic activities burn more fat than others in a given period of time, because they involve more-strenuous muscular participation than others. For example, it is obvious that one would burn more fat running than walking for an hour. The following chart will give you an idea of how much fat you (a woman of about 125 pounds) will burn in twenty minutes of activity. (If you weigh double that, you will burn one-third to double the amount of fat for that same twenty minutes.)

AEROBIC EXERCISE CHART

Aerobic Activity	Calories Burned per 20 Minutes
Bottoms Up! Workout (no rests)	315
Bottoms Up! Workout (with allowed rests)	265
Fat-Burning Workout	265
Stair machine	260
Running an eight-minute mile	230
Running a nine-minute mile	220
Cross-country skiing	220
Swimming	210
Stair stepping	200
Rope jumping	200
Low-impact aerobics (aerobic dance)	200
Nordic track machine	165
Trampoline jumping	165
Race walking	160
Hiking (hills)	150
Rowing machine	150
Jogging at easy pace	145
Bicycle riding	140
Moderate dance (freestyle)	120
Walking at fast pace	110

If you want to burn even more fat as you perform the above exercises, flex your muscles as you work. This added tension will cause your body to work harder and to burn additional fat. (Note that where pace is not indicated on the chart, a moderately brisk pace is assumed.) You can of course burn even more fat by speeding up the pace.

BREAKING IN GENTLY

If you are not already used to doing aerobics for twenty minutes or more, it's a good idea to start slowly. Follow this schedule, and use your own judgment in combination with the advice of your doctor on how to modify it according to your needs.

Week 1: three to five minutes
Week 2: five to seven minutes
Week 3: seven to ten minutes
Week 4: ten to fifteen minutes
Week 5: fifteen to twenty minutes
Week 6: twenty to twenty-five minutes
Week 7: twenty-five to thirty minutes
Week 8: thirty to thirty-five minutes
Week 9: thirty-five to forty minutes

Note: The above schedule does not apply to brisk walking. If you are not used to walking at all, walk for ten minutes a day the first week and increase it by five minutes per week until you are walking up to an hour a day.

You should work from the lower end of each week's range upward, so that by the end of the week you are at the higher end of the range. For example, on the first day of week one, you may run for three minutes. The next day you run, you may run for four minutes, and by the end of the week, you may run for five minutes. Then on week two you may start with five minutes and work your way up to seven minutes by the end of the week, and so on.

Don't be impatient. It's better to take it slow and avoid injury or fatigue. If you rush it, you may be tempted to be hard on yourself and to say things like "See. It's too much for you. Who are you trying to kid?" when you find yourself fatigued after an abusive aerobic session. In some cases it's better to take it slow and, in the end, to feel as if it was too easy. Better to go slow than to quit! The annoying break-in period will be ancient history in a matter of weeks, and you won't regret having taken the time to do it right.

WALKING, AS OPPOSED TO JOGGING OR RUNNING

When it comes to walking, as opposed to jogging or running, the same amount of fat can be burned—only you'll have to do it longer. Note, for example, that the chart indicates that you will burn 110 calories after twenty minutes of walking, but 220 calories after running at a decent pace (a nine-minute mile). So if you prefer walking fast over running, it will take you twice as long, but you will burn the same amount of fat—and perhaps more!

What? Do you actually burn more fat by going slower? Perhaps. Remember I said that the ideal fat-burning range is between 60 and 70 percent of capacity? The reason for this is due to the fact that it is the duration of the exercise rather than the intensity that makes for maximum fat burning, and when you're keeping your pulse in the 60 to 70 percent maximum range, you can go a much longer period of time without having to stop. In fact, most people can indeed walk for an hour or more.

How is fat burned during an aerobic exercise? In the initial stages of the exercise, glycogen is burned until that glycogen is used up. Then and only then do you start to burn fat—and continue to burn fat until you stop exercising. When you run, you may tire too soon to continue going long enough to burn as much fat as you would if you walked and were able to continue forever.

For maximum heart and lung capacity development, however, it is a good idea to get your heart rate up to about 80 percent of capacity. So if you enjoy the stair machine or running, and if your doctor says it's OK, go for it.

All of the above notwithstanding, many people choose walking over running because walking is comparatively easy on the joints and bones and can be done by people with osteoarthritis (deterioration of the joints). In fact, walking can help people with such a disease to gain strength to negotiate stairs and to eventually walk farther and with more vigor. Walking also helps to strengthen the entire body musculature, without the stress to bones and joints that running or high-impact aerobics can cause.

STEP AEROBICS.
AEROBIC DANCE AND STATIONARY BIKE

The newest rage in aerobic activity is step aerobics, a form of activity where a group of people step up and down onto various steps to the sound of music. It's easy to perform, and with the right instructor it's safe. It burns about the same amount of calories as does low-impact aerobics taken at a brisk pace. This activity is also fun because you get to enjoy the fellowship of "steppers"—a special combined energy is created by the group. You begin to have fun, and the time flies.

The disadvantage of step aerobics is that unless you want to do it alone at home (boring, because you are stepping up and down, up and down, and performing the exact same movement endlessly), you must spend travel time to get to the activity. If you are a busy person, this can be a problem.

Some people foolishly believe that step aerobics are sufficient to tighten and reshape the thigh and hip/buttock areas. It cannot. Step aerobics helps to strengthen these areas and helps to build endurance, but step aerobics can never sculpt the perfectly shaped muscles needed for the look most women seek. You have no choice but to work with weights the right way in order to achieve that goal.

Aerobic dance is an excellent choice for an aerobic activity. It provides fun and camaraderie, and in addition it stresses every muscle in the body for overall strength and endurance. If you do choose aerobic dance, be sure to choose low-impact aerobics as opposed to full-impact aerobics. The difference between the two is that with high-impact aerobics you do a lot of jumping and leaping—in other words, both feet leave the ground at the same time quite often in the workout. End result? Unsafe stress on bones and joints. With low-impact aerobics, both feet never leave the ground at the same time. End result? A well-balanced overall aerobic workout without the stress on bones or joints.

If you're anything like me, and are not especially well coordinated, you may prefer to ride your stationary bicycle while watching television, reading the paper, or listening to music or self-help tapes.

Even though you will have to ride the bike a little longer to burn the same amount of fat you would burn doing step aerobics or aerobic dance, it may be worth it, because at least the bike allows you to accomplish two things at once. In addition you'll save the travel time to and from the bench aerobics or aerobic dance class.

If you choose to ride the bike, set the tension at a very low range and enjoy rather than suffer the ride. Setting the tension low will ensure that you don't wear down your developing thigh muscles—and that you burn only fat. It will also make the workout most pleasant and allow you to go for a greater length of time.

If you wish, you can use one of those bikes that has an attachment for your upper body to stimulate your arms, chest, and back as you bike. I hate those devices and find that biking is no longer fun when I try to use them, but if you don't mind them, then all the better. You get total body stimulation, but remember to set the tension low or you may wear down hard-earned muscle.

STAIR MACHINES, ROWING MACHINES, AND NORDIC TRACK MACHINES

Stair machines, rowing machines, and Nordic track machines can be used either in the gym or in one's apartment. In either case they can be used while watching television, but not while reading (too much jolting—even if you were able to concoct a steady holding device).

Stair machines challenge the lower body: the thighs, hips, and buttocks. But don't be fooled into thinking that you can substitute this machine for a lower-body workout. The machine forces you to repeatedly move your lower body so that your muscles are developing an endurance ability. Muscles cannot, however, be sculpted and shaped by the stair stepper. In fact, you will have to work with the weights as described in this book to do that.

Rowing machines stress mainly the upper body: the chest, shoulders, back, biceps, and even triceps. Some lower body work is involved (your legs and buttocks are moving), but not as much as the upper body. Even with all of that, don't dream for a moment that you can substitute the rowing machine for the upper body workout described in this book. The rowing machine can help to build upper body strength and endurance, but it cannot sculpt perfectly formed muscles.

The Nordic track machine combines both upper and lower body work, and it is an excellent overall strength- and endurance-building device. But once again, such a machine can never be used as a substitute for a scientifically formulated, body-sculpting upper- and lower-body workout. If you choose any of these machines, be sure to set the tension as low as possible to prevent wearing down hard-earned muscles.

CROSS-COUNTRY SKIING, SWIMMING, ROPE JUMPING, AND TRAMPOLINE JUMPING

Although cross-country skiing is a sport, it is also an aerobic activity, because it keeps your heart rate well within the ideal fat-burning range for the twenty minutes or more that you are performing the activity. It is the steady, rhythmic pace of this activity that gives it its aerobic component. The entire musculature is involved in the workout; arms, shoulders, chest, back, stomach, hips, buttocks, and legs are working. It is enjoyable for those who like the outdoors and who don't mind a little cold weather—and what's more, it is easy to do and there's none of the danger of downhill skiing. It is unlikely that one would cross-country ski more than once a week, so if you choose this as your aerobic activity, you will naturally want to combine it with other choices.

If you like the water, swimming can be your aerobic activity of choice. It is especially appealing to those who have sustained various injuries and cannot afford even the slightest stress on the bones or joints. In fact, swimming helps to loosen stiff joints. The entire musculature is involved in swimming, with a special emphasis on the chest, shoulders, back, and abdominal muscles. If you choose swimming as your regular aerobic activity, keep in mind that there is swimming, and then there is *swimming*. If you are going to take it easy in the water and do side- or backstrokes that propel you for long distances and allow you to rest during that propulsion, you will of course not get as much calorie burning as you would if you did a straight crawl or the butterfly.

Rope jumping can be a life saver if you are away from home and want to keep your aerobic activity without leaving the privacy of your hotel or guest room. It has been my main aerobic activity when I am on the road and have minimum time to spare. I jump out of bed, splash cold water on my face, throw on an old T-shirt and shorts, and turn on the TV for the morning news. I look at the clock, and still half-asleep, I start jumping. Twenty minutes later, it's over. I take a shower and dress and I'm off. It was quick. It was painless. And I didn't waste one minute getting to or from a workout place or talking to people.

Rope jumping challenges all the muscles of the body because you have to swing the rope around and jump at the same time; you are forced to use your upper as well as your lower body muscles. Rope jumping is not the ideal activity for those with back, knee, or ankle problems because it does put some stress on the joints.

Trampoline jumping has all the benefits of rope jumping—if you move your arms while you're jumping—and it's more fun because taking advantage of the springs in the trampoline allows you to bound high into the air. True, you can't take a trampoline with you if you're traveling, but as far as equipment goes, it takes up very little space. It can be set on its side in even the smallest apartment, or shoved under the bed.

The best way to use the trampoline is to play your favorite music and then jump, march, dance, trot, or strut, as your mood dictates. You can swing your arms in accordance and have yourself a time. The best part of it all is this piece of equipment is so inexpensive that you can purchase one (see p. 284 to order one) and do it in the privacy of your own home—so no one will be able to report you to the authorities as you swing and leap wildly about. (I do this, and I often think "Thank God nobody can see me," and then I laugh wildly and continue to bounce away.)

RACEWALKING AND HIKING

Most of us have seen racewalkers. At first, they appear quite comical, because they seem to be walking in a quick, rigid, robotic fashion. But there is a method to their madness. They are positioning their bodies and timing the moves in order to achieve maximum speed without bouncing off the ground and breaking into a run.

Racewalking can be fun and, in fact, can net you a greater speed than moderate running or fast jogging. I'll never forget the time I tried to keep up with some racewalkers on a morning "walk" at a health spa. I ended up having to run at a moderate pace in order to keep up. There was no way I could keep from springing off the ground and still stay up with them.

Racewalking utilizes all of the body's muscles and is an excellent overall workout. It helps to strengthen and condition the muscles without wearing them down and without putting undue stress on the bones and joints.

Hiking at a fast pace along hilly terrain, especially if you love the outdoors, can be a near-spiritual experience. While enjoying the beauty of nature, you will at the same time challenge all of the muscles in the body, especially the lower hips, buttocks, thighs, and calves. You will increase muscle strength in those areas. People with knee or back problems may not be able to participate in hilly hikes and may have to settle for straight terrain. Some calorie burning will of course be sacrificed in this case.

Either racewalking or hiking can be used as a regular aerobic activity.

205

FAST SOCIAL DANCING

In order for social dancing to be considered an aerobic activity, it has to be performed for twenty minutes without stopping (except for changing partners or the momentary wait for the change of music). Dances that fit the aerobic category are disco, freestyle (where continuous vigorous movement is involved), latin (salsa, merengue, mambo, or any continuous-movement latin dance), quick-movement ballroom dancing, and so on.

Dancing involves all of the muscles of the body and usually does not put undue stress on the joints or bones. It's also a lot of fun. Rarely does one feel as if one is working while dancing. (The realization usually comes after the dancing, when you say to yourself, "Wow, I'm tired. I really worked out.")

Most people do not go out dancing three times a week, so if you choose dancing as your aerobic activity, you will have to combine it with other aerobic choices.

SPORTS—OR SEMI-AEROBIC ACTIVITIES THAT BURN FAT

If you are performing the Bottoms Up! Workout four or more days a week and you prefer to participate in a sport rather than an aerobic activity, you may do so. Sports such as tennis, racquetball, and even golf help you to burn fat. The more taxing the sport, of course, the more fat you will burn. Here is a chart that will give you an idea of how much fat you can expect to burn per twenty-minute session for certain sports.

SPORTS CHART

Sport	Calories Burned per 20 Minutes
Karate, judo	300
Racquetball	200
Squash	200
Handball	200
Waterskiing	180
Horseback riding	180
Rowing or canoeing	180
Roller- or ice-skating	180
Downhill skiing	180
Tennis (singles)	160
Tennis (doubles)	140
Volleyball	140
Frisbee	140
Golf	105

Sports such as the ones mentioned above have a fat-burning effect because they force the body to work hard—even though the activity is not sustained for twenty uninterrupted minutes.

If the above sports have a fat-burning effect, why should you care if they don't have an aerobic effect? Well, if you're doing the Bottoms Up! Workout or the Fat-Burning Workout, you don't have to worry about it much, because you are already getting quite an aerobic effect from the workout. As mentioned above, however, since short rest periods are allowed in those workouts (if you take advantage of them), it would be ideal if you also participated in a straight aerobic activity.

If your time is limited, however, and you enjoy a certain sport over any possible straight aerobic activity—even though, technically speaking, you cannot get an aerobic effect unless you work uninterrupted for twenty minutes—you can get a semi-aerobic effect. For example, if you are playing hard tennis nearly nonstop for seven minutes, you've gotten seven minutes' worth of aerobics, and your heart and lungs are strengthened more than they would be if you sat in a chair for that length of time.

Keep in mind also that some of the above sports (fast horseback riding, canoeing, and waterskiing, for example) can indeed be performed for twenty minutes or more nonstop and can then be considered straight aerobics.

OTHER NON- OR SEMI-AEROBIC ACTIVITIES THAT BURN FAT

You can burn a lot more fat by doing the daily work that is required of you around the house than you can by dozing on the couch. (You burn about 60 calories an hour sleeping, 80 calories an hour sitting in a chair and relaxing with a book, and about 95 calories an hour standing.)

When you are at home and are tempted to just "vegetate," remember the fat-burning effect of any kind of activity, and you may just decide to rake those leaves, weed that garden, trim those hedges, vacuum that floor, clean those windows, or shovel that snow. Here is a chart that depicts certain household activities.

HOUSEHOLD CHORES CHART

Activity	Calories Burned per 20 Minutes
Shoveling snow	250
Mowing the lawn	170
Trimming hedges	100
Weeding	95
Window cleaning	80
Mopping	75
Furniture polishing	75
Vacuuming	70
Raking	70
Light dusting	60

(If you are comparing the chart above to sleeping, sitting, or standing, remember that the figures mentioned in the above paragraph regarding these sedentary activities are calculated per hour, while the household-activity chart gives calories burned per 20 minutes. In other words, you burn about 20 calories in twenty minutes of sleeping on the couch, while you could have burned 60 calories in that twenty minutes if you got up off your —— and dusted the house.)

What happens if you weed the garden for ten minutes or shovel snow for only five? Just divide the number into twenty and you will see how much fat you burned for that period of time.

ANY ACTIVITY—FOR ANY PERIOD OF TIME— BURNS SOME FAT

What is the bottom line of fat burning? It's better to be awake than asleep. It's better to sit than to lie down. It's better to stand than to sit. It's better to walk than to stand. It's better to walk fast than to walk slow. It's better to sustain an activity for a longer period of time than for a shorter period of time. But in any case it's better to do something than to do nothing. The fact is, and always was, the more activity that you are involved in in a given day, the more fat you will burn.

A WORD ABOUT CALORIES AND FAT

As most of you already know by now, for every 3,500 calories that are in "deficit" in your body, your body must use up one pound of stored fat for energy in order to function. So the more calories you burn, of course, the more fat you burn.

HOW MUCH AEROBICS SHOULD YOU DO?

If you have the time, the ideal amount of aerobic activity is three to six 20- to 30-minute sessions per week. If you are bound and determined to lose all excess fat, you can perform an aerobic activity for ten days straight—and then you really should take a day off.

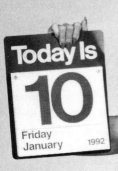

Today Is
10
Friday
January 1992

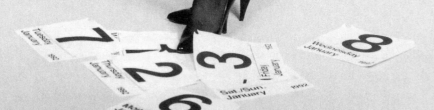

8
WEEKLY WORKOUT PLANS AND MAINTENANCE

A workout plan is vital to the success of your program. Whether you have minimum or maximum time to spend on your fitness regimen, it's a good idea to write out a weekly plan and to follow it so that your routine can quickly become a habit—something that you do without thinking and without negotiating the issue, like taking a shower or brushing your teeth.

Some people have very little time and want to know what they can do as a bare minimum to get in shape. Others are also very busy but have a little more time to invest, and they are able to do the regular Bottoms Up! Workout that calls for just the right amount of time. Others consider themselves to be fitness fanatics and/or are willing to work out as much as possible in order to get in shape as quickly as possible. Yet these people want to be sure that they are investing their workout minutes in the best possible way—so that they get maximum results without overtraining in any one area.

This chapter contains workout plans for each of the above and, in addition, provides maintenance plans so that you can stay in shape for the rest of your life without experiencing workout fatigue and without being bored to death.

211

BOTTOMS UP!—THE BARE MINIMUM PLAN

The bare minimum workout plan requires that you exercise your lower and middle body two days a week and your upper body two days a week. Here's how it looks in a weekly schedule:

Sunday	Monday	Tuesday	Wednesday	Thursday	Friday	Saturday
	Lower	Upper		Lower		Upper
	Middle			Middle		

As you will recall, your lower and middle body workout includes thighs, hips/buttocks, and abdominals. Your upper body workout includes chest-shoulders, biceps-triceps, and back-calves.

Your total time investment will be twenty to thirty minutes per workout, depending upon how fast you go and how many of the optional zero-to fifteen-second rests you take.

In review, if you follow the bare minimum plan, you will get this total workout:

Lower body: two times per week
Middle body: two times per week
Upper body: two times per week

I am allowing you to leave out regular aerobics, because the Bottoms Up! Workout has a built-in aerobic effect. If it comes down to it and you have only just so much time to exercise, it is vital that you work with the weights aerobically, as in this workout, instead of skipping the weights completely and just doing aerobics. Aerobics alone cannot reshape your body!

Suppose you can't fit your workout days in as above. Say, for example, you are just too busy during the heart of the work week to exercise, but your schedule allows you to work out toward the end of the week and on the weekends. No problem. You can do it. Of course it would be ideal to spread the workout evenly over your week, but if you can't, you will get excellent results anyway.

If you work out four days in a row and rest for three days, one of two things may happen during the three-day rest period: either your body will miss working out and haunt you to get back to it, or you'll be tempted not to start up again after three days off. If the latter is the case, you'll have to use self-discipline and just do it.

If all of your workout time is available toward the end of the week, here is how your plan may look. (Note that I have rearranged the calendar, with Monday at the beginning, to demonstrate this point.)

Monday	Tuesday	Wednesday	Thursday	Friday	Saturday	Sunday
			Lower	Upper	Lower	Upper
			Middle		Middle	

If you choose a plan such as above, you may forget which body parts you exercised last, so it is especially important for you to write out a weekly schedule.

What if you can only work out two or three days a week? Don't let this discourage you. Simply work out on those days, but remember: never exercise the same body parts two workout days in a row. In other words, if you exercised your lower and middle body the last time you worked out, and then didn't work out for five days, the next time you work out, make sure you exercise the upper body. Why? You don't want to create a lopsided body. No matter how often you work out, this rule holds true. You never work the same body part two days in a row. (The one exception is the abdominals. This will be discussed below, but it does not concern you unless you are interested in the regular or maximum workouts.)

BOTTOMS UP!—THE REGULAR PLAN

The regular workout plan requires that you exercise the lower body three days a week, the middle body four days a week, and the upper body two days a week, and that you do three sessions of aerobics per week. Here is a sample plan:

Sunday	Monday	Tuesday	Wednesday	Thursday	Friday	Saturday
Lower	Upper	Lower	Aerobics	Upper	Lower	Aerobics
Middle	Aerobics	Middle		Middle	Middle	

In review, if you follow the "regular," or ideal, plan, you will get this total workout:

Lower body: three times per week
Middle body: four times per week
Upper body: two times per week
Aerobics: three times per week

Why this particular combination? For the perfect health and fitness plan, in addition to even aerobic-type weight training, it's a good idea to include three sessions of regular aerobics per week. (See chapter 7 for a discussion on aerobics.) For optimum initial development of your stomach muscles, it is necessary to challenge that area at least four days a week. Later, when your stomach is in shape, you can switch to twice a week.

Why exercise the middle body four days a week and not the lower body? When it comes to workout frequency, the stomach stands alone among body parts. In order for fastest development, the stomach should be exercised four to six days a week.

The lower body needs lots of exercises—more exercises than the middle body—but the lower body does not have to be exercised more than two or three times a week. (You will note that I give seven exercises for each lower body part and five exercises for the abdominal area.) So you see, where number of exercises are concerned, the lower body needs more work, but when a frequency of exercise is concerned, the middle body needs more work.

What if you want to change the above specific workout days to suit your own needs? Of course you can do it, but here are some important rules:

1. **Never exercise the lower body two days in a row.** For optimum development your lower body muscles need forty-eight hours to rest before working again. If you ignore this rule, you are in danger of overtraining your thighs; and you may wear down hard-earned muscle. What can you do the day after you train lower body muscles? You may do the upper body workout and/or the middle body workout and/or an aerobic workout, or you may rest.

2. **Never exercise the upper body two days in a row.** For optimum development upper body muscles need forty-eight hours to rest before working again. If you ignore this rule, you are in danger of overtraining the upper body muscles and may wear down hard-earned muscle. What can you do the day after an upper body workout? You may do the lower and/or the middle body on the next workout day, you may do aerobics, or you can simply rest.

3. **The middle body (abdominals) can be exercised every day, any day**—no matter what else you are or are not exercising on that day. In other words, you can fit in an extra abdominal workout anytime, at your convenience.

4. **Aerobics can be done every day, any day**—no matter what else you are or are not exercising on that day. In other words, feel free to fit

aerobics into your workout schedule whenever it is convenient for you.

WORKING THE ENTIRE BODY ON ONE DAY

What if you want to exercise your entire body in one day, because you know you won't have time to do the other half of the body the next day, or because you skipped a workout the day before? You can do this if you have the energy. It will take you forty minutes to an hour.

If you dare the grueling workout of both the upper and the lower and middle body workouts in one day, remember to follow the rules above. On the next day you must rest both upper and lower body. You can do middle body work and/or aerobics the next day, or you can rest.

BOTTOMS UP!—THE MAXIMUM PLAN

If you are a woman who wants to speed up her progress and if you have the time and energy to invest and want to know exactly how to work out without overtraining, here is a plan for you:

Sunday	Monday	Tuesday	Wednesday	Thursday	Friday	Saturday
Aerobics	Upper	Lower	Upper	Lower	Upper	Lower
	Middle	Middle	Middle	Middle	Middle	Middle
	Aerobics	Aerobics	Aerobics	Aerobics		Aerobics

If you follow the maximum plan, you will get this workout:

> **Lower body:** three times per week
> **Middle body:** six times per week
> **Upper body:** three times per week
> **Aerobics:** six times per week

This is the ultimate plan. It will have you working out between twenty and forty minutes per session, and most days it will have you working out twice a day. Let me explain.

The upper body workout takes twenty to thirty minutes. The middle body workout takes about five to ten minutes. So when you exercise upper and middle body in a given session, you will have worked for twenty-five to forty minutes. If you are also doing aerobics on that day, you will be doing another twenty- to thirty-minute workout session (depending upon how long you want to do aerobics). If you are exercising the lower and middle body on a given day, you will have worked from twenty to thirty minutes, depending upon how fast you go. If you are also doing aerobics on that day, you will be doing another twenty- to thirty-minute workout session also.

CAN YOU DO BOTTOMS UP! AND AEROBICS IN ONE LONG SESSION?

The body responds best when workouts are spread more evenly over the day. In other words, the ideal way to exercise would be to do your Bottoms Up! Workout (whether it be the upper body alone, or upper and middle, or lower and middle) in one training session, and then to wait at least four hours before doing your aerobic workout. But, if this is not possible and if you have the energy, there is no reason why you can't plough right through and do your aerobics right after you do your Bottoms Up! Workout. (You will want to take at least a five- to ten-minute break between your Bottoms Up! Workout and your aerobic workout.) If you do decide to bomb away and get it all over with in one marathon session, you will be exercising for an hour or more, depending upon how fast you perform Bottoms Up! and how many minutes you decide to do aerobics. (You may, of course, choose to do your aerobic workout first— and your Bottoms Up! Workout immediately following.)

IS IT OK TO DO AEROBICS EVERY SINGLE DAY AND NEVER TAKE A REST?

No. Most people take one day off a week from aerobics in order to give the body a day to recuperate and to prevent injury. I find I can push it to ten days in a row, but then I must take a day off. My body as well as my mind tell me to "give it a break," and I do.

IS IT OK TO EXERCISE YOUR ABDOMINAL MUSCLES EVERY SINGLE DAY AND NEVER TAKE A REST?

No. When it comes to the stomach muscles, one day off a week is mandatory in order to prevent overtraining and the possible wearing down of hard-earned stomach muscle.

If you train your stomach muscles six days a week, by the seventh day you will be happy to rest those muscles. In fact, while I *have* met people who want to do aerobics every day without stopping, I have *never* yet met a person who wants to exercise his or her stomach muscles every day without taking one day off a week.

WHAT IF YOUR UPPER BODY NEEDS MORE WORK THAN YOUR LOWER BODY?

Suppose you are one of those rare women who needs more work on the upper body than the lower body? In addition to doing the Wild Woman or Terminator Workout for the upper body (see page 218), you can do extra upper-body workouts, but leave out the extra lower-body workout. If you do this, here is how your schedule may look:

Sunday	Monday	Tuesday	Wednesday	Thursday	Friday	Saturday
Upper	Lower	Upper	Middle	Lower	Upper	Aerobics
Middle	Middle	Aerobics	Aerobics	Middle		
Aerobics	Aerobics			Aerobics		

If you follow this plan, you will get this workout:

> **Lower body:** two times per week
> **Middle body:** four times per week
> **Upper body:** three times per week
> **Aerobics:** six times per week

Note: You can of course do only three, four, or five days of aerobic work instead of six.

WHAT IF YOU WANT A WILD WOMAN OR TERMINATOR UPPER BODY?

Suppose you need lots of work for your lower body and middle body and you are happy that you have found the Bottoms Up! Workout, which puts the emphasis on those body parts, but you would also like an extrahard, well-developed, clearly defined upper body—you know, "terminator" arms. If this is you, you can add in the exercises described in the upper body workout in chapter 6.

If you want a little more work, do the Wild Woman routine, which adds one exercise to each upper body part. If you want to do the maximum of work, then do the Terminator plan, adding two exercises to each upper body part. You can also do Wild Woman or Terminator routines for only selected upper body parts—those body parts that you want to further develop, like arms only, for example. (See chapter 6 for details.)

Wild Woman and Terminator upper-body workouts will not affect your workout days; they will simply add a small amount of time to your upper-body workout days, so there is no reason to make special schedules for them.

PUTTING IT ALL TOGETHER

Now that you know the basic rules of the minimum and maximum workout, it's time for you to make up your own workout schedule. Get a calendar and write in your weekly schedule. Do this at the beginning of each week.

Review the above workout plans and then decide what you are willing and able to do. If you are not sure, why not start out by doing the minimum plan, and then as time goes by and you become more and more excited about the program and the results you are getting, you can advance to the regular and perhaps even the maximum plan.

By way of review, if you are using the bare minimum Bottoms Up! Workout, your workout schedule may look something like this:

Sunday	Monday	Tuesday	Wednesday	Thursday	Friday	Saturday
	Lower Middle	Upper		Lower Middle		Upper

It's better to go slowly and to progress at a steady pace than to try to rush yourself and bite off more than you can chew. The last thing I want to see happen is your quitting the program in disgust. If you never did one more thing than the bare minimum workout, in six months' time you would see such dramatic changes in your body that you and your friends and family would not be able to believe it was possible.

WORKOUT BURNOUT—WHEN TO SWITCH TO ANOTHER PROGRAM

"Do I have to do this program for the rest of my life?" This is one of the inevitable questions women ask when they first start one of my workout regimens.

The answer is simple. No.

You don't have to do *this* program for the rest of your life, but you do have to do something for the rest of your life. In the following paragraphs you'll find out just what that something is, and you may be surprised to see that there is more variety than you imagined.

It's a good idea to change your workout once in a while in order to prevent workout burnout and to shock your body into making more progress. So even if you love the Bottoms Up! Workout and want to do it for the rest of your life, I suggest that after six months at the minimum, and a year or two at the maximum, you switch to one of the following plans. Then after three months to a year—or even two—you can switch back to Bottoms Up!

For Added Muscle Growth: Now or Never

If you want to build slightly larger muscles and are willing to work out with weights for forty-five minutes to an hour four days a week, the program in my book *Now or Never* is the one for you.

Now or Never offers a "regular" weight-training program in every sense of the word. You exercise one-half of your body on workout day one and the other half of your body on workout day two—just as you do in this program—*but* you work one body part at a time, and you rest between 30 and 45 seconds after each and every set, because you are using heavier weights.

The purpose of using heavier weights is to build slightly larger muscles—not the "Arnold" kind (for those you would have to exercise two hours a day six days a week and take steroids, a male hormone—something I've never done and certainly do not recommend.)

How will you know if you want to switch to *Now or Never*? After six months to a year of the Bottoms Up! Workout, take a hard look at your body. Do you want slightly bigger muscles? If you do, the only way you're going to get them is by working more slowly and with heavier weights. You can even use *Now or Never* selectively, to build certain body parts!

If you like working out in a gym, you will be especially pleased with *Now or Never*, because that book presents a full gym workout with all of the start and finish photographs for each and every gym exercise. (It also shows a fully illustrated home workout.)

You will burn a lot of fat when you work with *Now or Never*, and the workout will net you an additional permanent fat-burning element: slightly larger muscles that increase your metabolism so that you burn more fat all day and night—whether sleeping, standing, or sitting in a chair.

But the Now or Never Workout is not an aerobic workout, and it does not burn fat at the same speed as do the workouts in *The Fat-Burning Workout* and *Bottoms Up!* You'll have to do additional aerobics with the Now or Never Workout to get your heart and lungs into optimum condition and to burn additional fat.

After doing *Now or Never* for six months to a year, take another look at your body and see if you have added the amount of muscle size you want. If you have, you can switch back to Bottoms Up!, or you can switch to a workout that is similar to Bottoms Up! but at the same time quite different, the Fat-Burning Workout.

For Speed Fat-Burning and Muscle Shaping: The Fat-Burning Workout

The Fat-Burning Workout burns the same amount of fat as does Bottoms Up! (though you'll burn more fat with Bottoms Up! if you don't rest at all). Like Bottoms Up!, it is an aerobic routine as well as a body-shaping routine—but it is also very different from Bottoms Up! Let me explain.

With the routines in *The Fat-Burning Workout*, you exercise one body part at a time, but you do your first set of all of the exercises for that body part before you take a rest. In bodybuilding parlance, this is called "giant setting." You do one set of three to five exercises without stopping (depending upon which plan you choose—"Regular," "Intensity," or "Insanity"), and only then do you get a fifteen-second rest. I'll use the Insanity thigh routine to demonstrate how the program works.

There are five exercises in this routine: the squat, the lunge, the sissy squat, the front squat, and the leg curl. You do your first set of twelve repetitions for each of those exercises without resting. Then you rest fifteen seconds, and you pick up a slightly heavier weight and do your second set of ten repetitions for each of those exercises. You then rest another fifteen seconds, pick up a slightly heavier weight, and do you last set of eight repetitions for those exercises. You are finished with your thigh routine in record time. (The workout allows you the option of doing fifteen repetitions for each set.)

The Fat-Burning Workout forces you to work one muscle group to the maximum—nearly to fatigue—before it allows a rest. For some people this is a little too exhausting, and they find themselves having to take rests between sets. While this does not ruin the workout, it does cause slightly less fat burning. In contrast, the Bottoms Up! Workout asks you to exercise another body part while one body part is resting. This prevents muscle fatigue and takes away the temptation to rest where rests are not indicated.

Because with the Fat-Burning Workout you are working one muscle to the maximum without resting, the heaviness of the weights you can use is limited, and the muscle size you can achieve is also limited. With Bottoms Up!, on the other hand, since you are not working a muscle to exhaustion but rather switching back and forth between muscle groups, you can use heavier weights and, in turn, get slightly larger muscles—if you wish. (Of course, you can stay with lighter weights and keep your muscle-size development down to a minimum.)

Bottoms Up! concentrates more on the lower and middle body than does *The Fat-Burning Workout*. With the Bottoms Up! Workout, you do a required seven exercises for thighs and hips/buttocks, but with the Fat-Burning Workout you only do three required exercises for those body parts—with an additional two optional exercises. The stomach routine in *The Fat-Burning Workout* allows five exercises maximum, while the routine in *Bottoms Up!* allows six. Upper body routines in both books allow the same amount of work, but the work is done in a different manner.

Which workout is better? Both are extremely effective. The Fat-Burning Workout goes a little faster and gives a little more definition, but the Bottoms Up! Workout is not as exhausting and allows for building slightly larger muscles. It also bombs away at the lower and middle body. It is best not to stick with one workout forever. No matter how great the program, the human body craves change and will respond best when given a chance to do something different for a while; then, perhaps, you can go back to a favorite workout.

After doing the Bottoms Up! Workout for six months to a year, switch to the Fat-Burning Workout for a few months. If you like it, stay with it for a year, and then try Now or Never for a few months. Again, if you like it, stay with that a year. Then either go back to Bottoms Up! or the Fat-Burning Workout, or take a little vacation and do the 12-Minute Total-Body Workout for a while. I am constantly switching among these workouts.

Additional Hardness and Definition: The 12-Minute Total-Body Workout

The program in *The 12-Minute Total-Body Workout* requires only one set of three-pound dumbbells and only twelve minutes daily. It is very intense: you'll be sweating after four minutes because instead of using weights in the regular fashion, you will be using three-pound dumbbells and squeezing as hard as you can throughout the movements. You will create as much pressure as you can by continually flexing your muscles, even on the stretch part of the exercise (this sort of pressure is known as "dynamic tension").

The 12-Minute Total-Body Workout combines the secrets of bodybuilding with those of the martial arts. (I studied the martial arts for seven years: jujitsu, karate, and judo.) By moving the weights in the same manner as bodybuilders—and squeezing your muscles as hard as possible, the way martial artists do when they perform their *kata* (dancelike practice of punching and blocking movements)—you get muscles that are as hard as a rock with maximum definition. You cannot put on significant muscle size with this program, because you are using only three-pound dumbbells, but you do sculpt highly condensed (hard) muscles with maximum definition.

The best part of the program is that you do it the moment you get out of bed. You need no equipment but the three-pound dumbbells (you can purchase the three-pound waterweights for traveling). Bench presses and flyes are performed at the edge of a chair, sofa, or bed. You can truly do this exercise anywhere in the world. You can even do the workout with no dumbbells or waterweights at all, because you can create all the tension with your own squeezing.

I switch to this workout for weeks at a time when I am burned out and sick of exercising, or when I am on the road and have no choice. Amazingly, when I get back to one of my other workouts, I feel no aches and pains the next day. This proves to me that the twelve-minute program has indeed challenged my muscles. Before I invented it, I would stop working out completely for weeks at a time, and when I got back to my regular routine, I couldn't move, much less walk, the next day.

The 12-Minute Total-Body Workout also has detailed instructions on what to order from hotel menus—room service included—and how to eat out in restaurants and when on the run.

If you want to switch to the 12-Minute Total-Body Workout just for a change, you can do it for three months and then go back to one of the above plans. If your life has become too busy to do anything else, you could—believe it or not—remain with this plan forever, and you would not get out of shape. I have hundreds of letters from women who do nothing else but this program and who are thrilled with the results.

Ideally, if you have the time and energy, you should continue to change your routine at least every year or two and switch back and forth from *Bottoms Up!* to *Now or Never* and/or *The Fat-Burning Workout*—and where needed, to *The 12-Minute Total-Body Workout*.

CAN YOU HAVE A COMPLETE VACATION FROM WORKING OUT?

Good news. Yes. Every six months you can take a week off. I don't recommend taking two weeks off, because this is too long a time to let your muscles lie stagnant. What's more, there is no excuse for this because you can use the twelve-minute plan anywhere in the world.

If you do take a week off, it's not a good idea to completely vegetate for that week. Be active in other ways: walk, play a sport—do some mild form of exercise. Otherwise, your body will begin to feel sluggish.

You should take a week off from working with weights at least one week per year. The body needs a rest from muscle training in order to appreciate the workout fully. In fact, you will find that after taking a week off, your body will "jump" into better shape than ever before after three weeks of training again. It is almost as if the body is saying, "Thank you for letting me rest. But thank you more for letting me start again. I was afraid that you were going to let me lie stagnant, and I'm going to make sure that I make the most of the opportunity, now that you're letting me work out again."

A LIFETIME OF FITNESS

As I said above, No, you don't have to do Bottoms Up! for the rest of your life, but yes, you do have to do one of the above workouts for the rest of your life if you want to be in top shape forever. Experiment with each of the programs. You may find that you like one more than the others, and you may want to "major" in that one—using it for a year or so and then switching to another program for only three to six months for a change, and then switching back to your favorite program for another year or two.

You be the judge. After a while you will be more of an expert than I am as to just what is right for your body. That's how it works. You learn your own body, and as you decide what your goals for your body are, you will know what to do and when to do it.

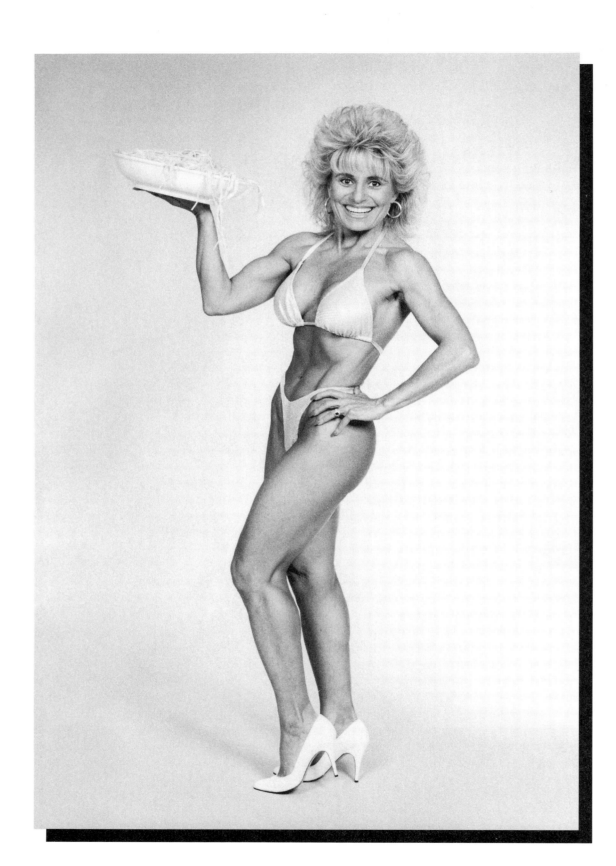

9

HOW TO EAT PLENTY AND LOSE FAT!

Working out is half the battle; eating right is the other half. Fortunately, eating right is a lot less difficult than most people realize. All you have to do is follow a few simple rules, and you can eat to your heart's content. You need never go hungry.

In the following pages you will learn the basics about food and how food is handled by the body. Once you read and understand these principles, right eating will become second nature to you. You won't have to memorize anything. If you need to, you can always skim through this chapter again for a quick reminder.

CALORIES—WHAT THEY ARE AND WHY YOU DON'T HAVE TO COUNT THEM IF YOU FOLLOW THIS EATING PLAN

A calorie is a unit of chemical energy released to your body when food is digested. In order to sustain life, the body must consume a certain number of calories every day.

You burn calories twenty-four hours a day, even in your sleep (about 60 calories an hour if your body is composed of a great deal of fat, and about 80 calories an hour if your body has a higher muscle-to-fat ratio).

In order to lose one pound of fat, you must create a calorie deficit of 3,500 calories. You can do this by taking in less calories than you need in a given day, by eating less, and by exercising and being generally physically active. The less calories you consume and the more energy you expend, the greater the calorie deficit you will create, and the more weight (pounds of stored fat) you will lose. But can you do this without counting calories?

If you follow the basic eating guidelines outlined in this chapter, you *will* keep your calories below the deficit line. That's because the unlimited complex carbohydrates I allow you are too low in calories to become a problem, and higher-calorie foods are limited. You won't have to count calories except, if you wish, to do a spot-check every so often. I have done all of the work for you. I will tell you which fatty foods to avoid completely, how to control your intake of simple sugars, and how much of allowed, nutritious foods you can eat. Your daily caloric intake will usually be between 1,500 and 2,000, but you won't have to check if you follow the eating guidelines in this chapter.

Some Calories Are Fatter Than Others

When you reduce the amount of fat in your diet, you reduce the number of calories you consume—in multiple. Let me explain. There are only 4 calories per gram of carbohydrates and protein, but there are 9 calories per gram of fat. So for every gram of fat you eliminate from your diet, you get double the benefit in terms of weight loss that you get for every gram of protein or carbohydrates that you eliminate from your diet. But there's more to it than that. The multiple-reduction benefit continues.

When you consume fat, only 2 to 3 percent of that fat is used up in the digestive process, but when you consume protein or carbohydrates, 20 to 25 percent of the calories are used up in the digestive process. How does this translate into your daily calorie intake? If you consume 1,000 calories in fat, about 980 of those calories are available to be used as energy or stored fat, but if you consume 1,000 calories in carbohydrates or protein, only about 750 of those calories are available for use as energy or stored fat.

The Bottoms Up! Eating Plan allows you to consume 20 to 25 grams of fat per day. Actually, even if you consumed 30 grams of fat a day, you would lose plenty of weight, but I want you to lose as fast as possible, so I'm asking you to keep your fat intake very very low.

Can You Eat As Much As You Want—As Long As You Keep the Fat Grams Low?

I recently spoke to a man who couldn't wait to tell me that he had actually gained weight, even though he was sticking to strictly low-fat foods. Gloating over the fact that he had proven the experts wrong, he bragged, "I never eat more than thirty grams of fat a day—yet I gained weight." At first I was surprised, but when I questioned him further, I discovered, as you might have guessed, that he overindulged in low- or nonfat foods full of simple, refined sugars. In other words, he was eating gallons of nonfat ice cream, and tons of low-fat cakes and puddings. He had brought his daily calorie intake so high that he was not able to burn those calories off in a given day. Of course he gained weight.

You won't have to worry about this happening to you if you follow the basic eating guidelines put forth in this chapter, because your intake of nonfat food products that contain simple sugars will be discouraged—and limited to three servings per week if you do decide to indulge.

Why You Must Limit Your Intake of Refined Sugar

I'm not going to tell you to completely eliminate foods with refined sugars from your diet. Unlike many other diets, the Bottoms Up! program allows you to indulge in an occasional tablespoon of jam or jelly, or some sugary hard candy, or a high-sugar, nonfat dessert. But you must limit your intake of these to three servings per week. One serving constitutes two teaspoons of jam or jelly, or seven pieces of hard candy, or whatever amount is considered "one serving" on the package of nonfat cake, cookies, or ice cream. There are two reasons why you must limit your intake of refined sugars.

First, they can hinder the burning of fat. When you consume an excessive amount of refined sugars, a large amount of glucose is released into your bloodstream. This causes your body to produce high levels of insulin, which inhibits hormone-sensitive lipase, the enzyme that is responsible for draining fat from the fat cells. This causes the body to stubbornly cling to its fat cells. In other words, when excessive insulin is produced by the body, fat cells are locked into the body. Your goal is to get rid of fat, not to lock it in—so of course you must limit your intake of refined sugars.

Second, they can stimulate your appetite. The overproduction of insulin caused by the overconsumption of refined sugars causes blood sugar to go directly to the liver, creating a deficit of blood sugar in the circulatory system. When this happens, a feeling of fatigue is experienced, and this is interpreted by the body as hunger. You will be tempted to keep going back for more and more food, and if you do this, you will, during the course of the day, eat more calories than you burn, creating a calorie excess instead of a calorie deficit. That excess will be stored as fat! You will have defeated your purpose.

I can imagine what you must be thinking right now. "I'm never going to eat anything with refined sugar again." Fine. That would be great. But if you do want to indulge in an occasional refined-sugar treat, you can do it, but you'll have to resist the temptation to keep going back for more. If you know that you are the type who will consume two jars of jam by the end of the day if you have that first tablespoon, then stay away from jam altogether. The 18 calories per teaspoon would be harmless if you left it at that and if it prevented you from indulging in a high-fat treat such as a doughnut—but not if you're going to eat two jars of jam at a sitting.

FAT

Fat is a necessary part of the diet. Our cell membranes and sex hormones are composed of fat, and our internal organs are protected by the surrounding fat that cushions them. Fat helps the body to absorb and make use of calcium and vitamins D, E, A, and K. The fact is we do need a certain amount of fat in our diet in order to maintain good health.

When it comes to the American diet, however, fat deficiency is not the problem. Even those people who follow seemingly nonfat diets manage to consume a healthy minimum of fat (the bare minimum of fat one should consume is about 10 percent of total calorie intake—or about 14 grams of fat). The Bottoms Up! Eating Plan suggests a minimum of 15 percent or 20 to 25 grams of fat. The average American consumes up to 85 grams of fat per day, which account for 50 percent of total caloric intake, and those on the high end of the scale consume more than 100 grams.

Some Fats Are Worse Than Others Health-wise, but All Fats Will Make You Fat!

If you are anything like me, your main reason for wanting to limit the fat in your diet is for beauty, or "vanity" purposes. You know that excessive fat is bad for your health, but if you are honest, your main concern is your appearance. You probably feel this way, as I do, because up until now, excessive fat may not have caused you health problems. But it can.

Let's face it. Health is important. If we consume too much fat, especially the wrong kinds of fat, we are in danger of heart failure. Either **saturated fats** or **unsaturated fats** will make you fat, but one is worse than the other when it comes to potential heart failure.

Saturated fats are the "bad guys" of this group because they raise your blood cholesterol. They are found mainly in animal products such as meat, milk, cheese, and butter and in coconut oil; except for coconut oil these fats become solid at room temperature.

Unsaturated fats are fatty acids that are liquid in form and are derived from nuts, seeds, and vegetables. They do not raise your blood cholesterol levels and, in turn, do not clog arteries or cause heart problems—but they do make you fat, just as fat as you get if you eat unhealthy, artery-clogging saturated fat.

If you follow the eating plan outlined in this chapter, you won't have to worry too much about which fat you are eating, because all pure fats and the foods that are high in fats are forbidden anyway.

What Is Cholesterol?

Cholesterol is a fatlike substance that has no calories. It helps to form the sex and adrenal hormones, vitamin D, and bile. It is also a component of cell membranes and nerve linings and is found in the brain, liver, and blood.

We don't have to consume cholesterol in order to survive, because the body naturally produces all of the cholesterol it needs.

It is the cholesterol found in the blood that can cause problems. When there is too much of a certain kind of cholesterol in the blood—LDL cholesterol, which has come to be labeled "bad" cholesterol—problems arise.

What Is the Difference Between Good Cholesterol and Bad Cholesterol?

Both HDL (good cholesterol) and LDL (bad cholesterol) are composed of lipoproteins, which are molecular structures made of fats (lipids) and proteins bonded together. These little packets travel through the bloodstream.

The LDL packet functions to carry cholesterol from its place of synthesis to cell membranes, where it is needed for maintenance of the cells. In addition, however, LDL carries cholesterol through the arterial walls. If an overabundance of LDL is carried through the arterial walls, it will eventually become deposited on the arterial walls as plaque. In such cases the arterial walls eventually become too narrow to allow blood to freely pass through them, and undue pressure is put upon the heart until heart failure or a host of other less detrimental heart-related problems occur.

HDL is called good cholesterol because it removes cholesterol from the bloodstream and helps transport it (LDL) out of the cells, into the bile, and into the intestines, where it is eventually excreted out of the body.

How Do You Know If You Have Too Much "Bad" Cholesterol?

At one time people falsely believed that as long as their overall cholesterol level was under 200, they could forget about being concerned with cholesterol. They also assumed that if their cholesterol level was over 200, they were in serious trouble. Today we know that it's not that simple. The person with the lower count can in fact be in more trouble than the person with the higher count, depending upon the ratio of HDL (good cholesterol) to LDL (bad cholesterol). In other words, it is not the total cholesterol count that is most important, but rather the ratio of total cholesterol to HDL.

To find out your ratio of total cholesterol to HDL, have your doctor perform a "fractionated" cholesterol test. This test measures your HDL against your LDL. The doctor then prepares a ratio, or an index. The lower your index, the lower your risk (an index of 4 or lower is considered low risk). For example, if your total cholesterol level is 200, and your HDL is 50, your index is 4 (50 goes into 200 four times). If on the other hand, your total cholesterol level is 200, but your HDL level is only

25, you are at great risk, because your index is 8 (25 goes into 200 eight times.)

HDL levels can be raised through regular exercise, such as the program described in this book. LDL can be lowered by keeping saturated fats low and eliminating smoking, alcohol, refined sugars, and caffeine.

Fat "Nevers" Until You Reach Your Goal

While you are trying to lose fat, there are certain foods that are composed of all fat, or nearly all fat, which should be completely avoided until you reach your goal: butter, margarine, lard, chicken fat, mayonnaise, sour cream, cream cheese, cheese of any kind, oil of any kind, bacon, beef, lamb, veal, all fried foods, all nuts and seeds, olives, avocados, and chocolate.

And by the way, in case you were wondering, margarine has just as many fat grams, spoon for spoon, as does butter, although margarine is thought to be better for your health because it is, for the most part, composed of unsaturated fats.

Fat Choices

You will not choose a specific "fat" as a choice for each day, the way you will choose two or three proteins, three to five limited carbohydrates, and two or three fruits. Instead, you will diligently watch to see that you have consumed no more than 20 to 25 grams of fat per day. As mentioned above, nearly every food contains some fat, especially the protein choices, so have no fear. You will not have a problem filling your fat allowance for the day, but just in case by some miracle you do—great. You are allowed to go under it. (Please write to me if you do. I want to put you in "Vedral's Believe It or Not!")

PROTEIN

Protein is used by the body to build tissue and to heal and repair the muscles and bones as well as the hair, fingernails, skin, ligaments, enzymes, blood, immune cells, and internal organs. In addition, protein plays a role in regulating the acid–alkaline balance of the blood and tissues, as well as the body's water balance. Protein is an essential element in the production of hormones, which control metabolism, growth, and sexual development.

When protein is digested, it is broken down into smaller units called amino acids. The body needs twenty-two amino acids to make the protein usable to the human body. The human body can manufacture all but eight of these units without the aid of an outside source. But to produce the other eight, which have come to be called essential amino acids, the body must be supplied with fish, poultry, beef, egg whites, yogurt, or legumes such as lentils, split peas, or beans.

Daily Protein Intake

Unlike fat, protein cannot be stored, so we must feed our body a small amount of protein at a time. A bare minimum of protein is 44 grams per day. Since you will be building muscle with this program, you will be allowed to eat more than that (people who work with weights can consume up to ½ gram daily per pound of body weight).

For example, if you weigh 120 pounds, you can consume about 60 grams of protein per day. If your doctor advises that you keep your protein consumption as low as 44 grams per day, such as is recommended for women by the Pritikin Longevity Center, that is fine with me. You will still be well within the limits of good health. The meal plans at the end of this chapter range between 45 and 65 grams of protein per day.

If you consume 60 grams of protein a day, you will have consumed 260 calories in protein (4 calories per gram of protein). Taking it a step further, since you will be eating about 1,800 to 2,000 calories with this program, protein intake will account for about 13 to 15 percent of total calories. This is a good balance. You will consume the rest of your calories in fat (13 to 14 percent) and carbohydrates (71 to 74 percent).

How to Avoid Fat When Eating Protein

In selecting your protein source, you will have to be careful to avoid "fat traps." For example, look at this:

FAT IN FAST-FOOD CHICKEN

4 Ounces of Fast-food Fried Chicken	Fat Grams
Drumstick	16
Thigh	19
Breast	15

Compare the above with the notorious fatty red meats:

4 Ounces of Broiled Beef, Lamb, or Veal	Fat Grams
Eye of round	7
London broil	7
Pot roast	10
Top sirloin	11
Filet mignon	12
Leg of lamb	10
Lamb loin chop	12
Lamb shoulder	13
Leg of veal	4
Veal loin chop	9
Veal shoulder roast	9
Pork tenderloin	6
Pork center loin	10
Fresh ham	13

If you're going to fry chicken and eat it fried and with the skin, you might as well eat red meats such as beef, lamb, veal, or pork! If you look at the chart, fried chicken with the skin contains more fat than any of these high-fat foods.

My point, of course, is not to encourage you to do just that, but rather to shock you into realizing that you must never eat fried poultry and that you must always remove the skin.

Look what happens when you cook chicken or turkey the right way— broiled, poached, boiled, or baked with no fat and with skin removed. There are about five grams of protein for each ounce of poultry or fish.

FAT IN SKINLESS CHICKEN (NOT FRIED)

4 Ounces of Skinless Chicken	Fat Grams
Chicken breast	5
Chicken drumstick	8

Turkey, cooked the same way, is even lower in fat!

FAT IN SKINLESS TURKEY (NOT FRIED)

4 Ounces of Skinless Turkey	Fat Grams
Turkey breast	2
Turkey leg	4

Another source of low-fat protein is fish.

FAT IN FISH

4 Ounces of Fish	Fat Grams
Haddock	0.05
Red snapper	0.5
Cod	0.6
Abalone	0.6
Sea bass	1.0
Flounder	1.6
Sole	1.6
Squid	1.8
Tuna in water	2.0
Pike	2.0
Halibut	2.4
Scallops	2.8
Brook trout	4.2
Salmon	7.4
Swordfish	8.0

Why Not Cheese?

Cheese is a source of protein, as well as a source of calcium, but even the lowest of the low-fat brands are too high in fat to be allowed on a fat-loss diet. The best thing you can do for yourself is to forget all about cheese until you reach your weight goal.

FAT IN CHEESE

1 Ounce Regular Cheese	Fat Grams
Feta	6.0
Mozzarella	6.1
Jarlsberg	6.9
Provolone	7.6
Limberger	7.7
Gouda	7.8
Swiss	7.8
Edam	7.9
Muenster	8.5
Monterey Jack	8.6
Roquefort	8.7
Processed American	8.9
Colby	9.1
Cheddar	9.4

Just think of it. One little slice of cheese uses up almost half of your allowed fat grams for the day. And if you're in a snacking mood, you can stand at the refrigerator with the door open and consume at least three or four slices and think nothing of it. In fact, such nibbling will not even "register" as eating, and an hour later, you can eat a regular meal. See how insidious fatty foods are? But if you instead picked at a bowl of fresh strawberries, no harm would be done. You would feel full and would have consumed zero fat grams!

What about low-fat cheese? It is true that low-fat cheeses are much lower in fat than regular cheese, but they are really still too high for this program because one slice is rather high in fat anyway—and one slice is rarely enough to satisfy your cheese urge.

FAT IN LOW-FAT CHEESE

1 Ounce of Low-Fat Cheese	Fat Grams
Reduced-calorie American	2.2
Lite cheddar	3
Lite Swiss	3
Part-skim mozzarella	4.5

What About Cottage Cheese?

Cottage cheese is in a different category than sliced cheese. If you eat very low-fat or nonfat cottage cheese, you will not overstep your daily fat allowance. Here is a list of fat content for cottage cheese, ranging from full fat to nonfat.

FAT IN COTTAGE CHEESE

One-Half Cup of Cottage Cheese	Fat Grams
Nonfat brand	
1 percent fat	0
2 percent fat	1.2
Creamed or 4 percent fat	2.2
	5.1

Vegetarian Sources of Low-Fat Protein

There is plenty of protein in low-fat yogurt (17 grams per cup), beans (10 grams per cup), skim milk (8 grams per cup), tofu (7.8 grams in 3.5 ounces), and egg whites (4 grams in a large egg white). If you are a vegetarian, you can live on these proteins in combination with rice and corn and do just fine without ever eating meat again.

Two to Three Protein Choices per Day

When choosing your protein servings for the day, you may select from the above low-fat choices. You may have two protein choices a day: 6 ounces of fish, chicken, or turkey; 1 cup of skim milk; ⅔ cup of low-fat cottage cheese; 1 cup of low-fat yogurt; ½ cup of any beans or tofu.

Nonfat Food Products

It is usually best to choose a nonfat food over a food with even a trace of fat—*if.* And here is the big IF: if you are not going to abuse the eating of nonfat foods to the point where you consume so many calories in a given day that you end up eating, say, 3,000 calories a day. Let me explain.

Simplesse, the new wonder substitute for fat, which is made of the proteins from egg whites in combination with nonfat milk products, is now used in cottage cheese. Just because the cottage cheese is nonfat does not mean that you are allowed to eat limitless amounts of it. You must still count a ⅔-cup serving of that product as one protein serving for the day.

CARBOHYDRATES

Carbohydrates include many foods, and they break into two categories: simple carbohydrates and complex carbohydrates. Simple carbohydrates are sugars which themselves break down into two groups: refined and unrefined. Sugars in candy and cake are refined; sugars in fruit are unrefined. Complex carbohydrates include vegetables, grains, and fiber. Both simple and complex carbohydrates are the main source of energy to the body and the brain.

Complex carbohydrates are best for a gradually released source of energy. Simple, unrefined carbohydrates such as fruits are good for immediate energy.

Fruits Are Simple Sugars, Too—But!

Even though fruits are not refined sugars, they are still simple sugars and are converted into glucose (potential energy) quickly—more quickly than complex carbohydrates. Like refined sugars, fruits give a quick energy boost, followed by a drop in energy if you eat them on an empty stomach. Still, they are better than simple refined sugars, which do the same thing, because fruits contain fiber and vitamins and because the sugar in a fruit is not as concentrated as the sugar in, say, a candy bar. In other words, you would have to eat three pieces of fruit to consume the equivalent of the simple sugar found in one candy bar.

Two or Three Fruit Choices

For your fruit treat you may choose among all the fruits available. Each of the following fruits will count as one fruit serving:

large apple	1 large orange
4 apricots	1 cup papaya
small banana	1 large peach
1 cup berries (any kind)	1 medium pear
½ cantaloupe	3 persimmons
15 large cherries	¼ large pineapple
½ grapefruit	½ large plantain
20 grapes	2 plums
¼ honeydew melon	3 fresh prunes
large kiwi	1½ cups strawberries
3 kumquats	2 tangerines
1 small mango	1½ cups watermelon
1 large nectarine	

You may indulge in other fruit not listed here. Use your own judgment as to how much of that fruit constitutes a serving.

Complex Carbohydrates—and Low Caloric Density

Recent research has proven what should have been obvious to us all, but I must confess I never thought about it before now. If you eat a food that weighs more than another food but has the same amount of calories, you will have to eat less food to feel full, and in the end you will be able to consume less calories and lose more weight. Let's look into this further.

Caloric density refers to the number of calories per weight of that particular food. Since the human stomach can hold a maximum of two to three pounds of food, if you eat potatoes and other heavy vegetables, you won't have to eat very many calories before your stomach is completely full and literally cannot hold any more food. On the other hand, if you try to fill up on other, lighter-weight complex carbohydrates, such as whole wheat bread or dried cereals, be they ever so nutritious, you will have to consume many more calories in order to feel full.

Let's be more specific. If you eat one large baked potato weighing 8 ounces, one cup each of green beans, acorn squash, and broccoli, you will have eaten two pounds of food and will have consumed only 400 calories. Your stomach will be full and you will feel stuffed. To get the same full feeling on whole wheat bread, however, you will have to consume two pounds and 1,800 calories. To fill up on dry cereal would cost you even more calories: two pounds would amount to more than 3,000 calories.

What am I saying—that you should not eat whole wheat bread and dry cereal? Of course not. In fact, you must schedule these foods into your weekly meal plan for nutrition and variety, but if you are really feeling hungry and want to feel full and satisfied quickly, remember the low-caloric-high density trick.

The following is a list of low-density, low-calorie foods that are the best calorie bargain for filling you up.

Most unlimited complex carbohydrates (see pages 243 and 244)
Vegetables of every kind (potatoes, sweet potatoes, and yams are especially filling)
Whole grain pastas
Whole grains and brown rice
Oatmeal and other hot cereals

The caloric-density principle holds true for simple sugars, too. You will feel more full if you eat a pint of strawberries than if you eat two tablespoons of jelly. The strawberries will have one-fourth the calories of the jelly, and in the bargain you will have gotten plenty of fiber and vitamins from the strawberries—and not as much of an insulin burst, with all of its potential problems.

Three to Five Limited Complex Carbohydrates per Day

Each of the following constitutes one serving:

½ cup beans or lentils of any kind
1 cup corn or 1 large ear of corn
1 cup peas of any kind
1 large potato, sweet potato, or yam
1 cup winter squash

Each of the following whole grain, wheat, buckwheat, rye, cornmeal, oat, or sourdough products constitutes one serving:

½ bagel (the condensed kind; the light, airy ones count a whole bagel for
    one serving)
2 slices bread
1 ounce dry or hot cereals (measured uncooked)
8 crackers
1 English muffin
4 ounces pasta (measured dry)
2 ounces pretzels
¾ cup rice
4 rice cakes

Can you ever eat "white" or "refined" versions of the above? Yes, on occasion. But in general, stick to the healthier whole-grain wheat, buckwheat, rye, cornmeal, oat, or sourdough products.

Unlimited Complex Carbohydrates to Be Eaten Whenever You Are Hungry

You can feast on certain foods anytime, anywhere, and in any amounts. Really. I'm not kidding. Most vegetables fall into this category, with the exception of a few that I have listed above in the limited category. You should in fact consume a minimum of two and a half cups of unlimited complex carbohydrates per day. (This minimum is now recommended by the FDA. It may include corn, beans, peas, potatoes, and winter squash, counted in my limited category above.)

Asparagus	Kale
Beans, green or yellow	Leeks
Broccoli	Lettuce
Brussels sprouts	Mushrooms
Cabbage	Okra
Carrots	Onions
Celery	Peppers, red or green
Chickory	Radishes
Chinese cabbage	Rhubarb
Collard greens	Rutabagas
Cucumber	Shallots
Eggplant	Spinach
Endive	Sprouts
Escarole	Squash, zucchini or summer
Jerusalem artichoke	Tomatoes

FIBER

You will get your fiber from foods that are in the complex carbohydrates category. There are two types of fiber: soluble fiber, which can be digested by the body (found in oat bran, psyllium, fresh fruits, and vegetables and legumes); and insoluble fiber, which cannot be digested by the body (found in whole wheat, whole grains, celery, corn, corn bran, green beans, green leafy vegetables, potato skins, and brown rice).

We need a generous supply of soluble fiber in order to help lower blood sugar (soluble fiber slows down the body's absorption of carbohydrates and prevents an inordinate rush of insulin). Soluble fiber also helps to lower cholesterol levels by connecting with bile acids and escorting the cholesterol out of the body.

Insoluble fiber cannot be digested by the human body, so it is eliminated in the stool, supplying the stool with needed volume to help prevent constipation and colon and rectal cancer. But insoluble fiber has another wonderful benefit.

The Fat Vacuum!

Insoluble fiber helps to move the fat out of the body. Because insoluble fiber cannot be digested by the human body, it passes through the digestive track, and on its way it pulls some fat along with it. The fiber and the fat are then both eliminated in the stool.

Where's the Fiber?

The recommended daily allowance (RDA) for total fiber, as stipulated by the United States government, is about 30 grams per day. Here are the fiber counts for some foods.

FIBER COUNTS

Grains	Grams Fiber
1 ounce bran-flakes-type cereal	9
1 slice whole wheat bread	2
1 slice cracked wheat bread	2
1 slice rye bread	1
(In contrast, a slice of white bread has only ½ gram of fiber.)	

Fresh Fruits	Grams Fiber
1 orange	5
1 pear	5
1 cup of strawberries	5
1 banana	4
1 apple	3.5

Fresh Vegetables (1 cup each)	Grams Fiber
Spinach	11
Peas	8
Corn	8
Broccoli	8
Baked potato	6
Carrots	5
Eggplant	5
Green beans	5
Cabbage	4
Tomato	4

Beans and Legumes (1 cup each)	Grams Fiber
Baked beans	21
Split peas	21
Lentils	18

VITAMINS AND MINERALS

Vitamins are organic chemicals found in foods. Minerals are nutrients found in organic and inorganic combinations, and are needed in much greater amounts by the body than vitamins. Deficiency in various minerals can result in bone disease and in problems with the organs and the nervous system. If you eat a variety of the foods suggested in the complex carbohydrate category, fresh fruits, as well as a daily minimum of low-fat protein, you will get a full supply of vitamins and minerals.

It's much better to get your vitamins and minerals naturally than to depend upon food supplements—*i.e.,* pills. In fact, recent studies show that taking megadoses of vitamin and mineral supplements can cause an imbalance in the digestive system and prevent the body from absorbing the vitamins and minerals found in actual foods. I do not take any vitamins or food supplements, but I am not against them. You do what you and your doctor think is best for you.

How Much Calcium Do Women Really Need?

Calcium is the mineral largely responsible for keeping bones strong and healthy. A calcium deficiency can cause broken or brittle bones, especially as women pass the age of thirty. However, we now know that lack of calcium in the diet is not the only reason for thinning bones. Lack of weight-bearing exercise is as much a culprit. This workout will take care of that!

As far as diet goes, it is still a good idea to eat foods that keep you well within the recommended daily minimum of calcium, and to drink skim milk, which helps your body to utilize the calcium you consume by absorbing it into the bloodstream. (You can put skim milk in your coffee or tea, or on cold cereal.)

The RDA for calcium is 800 to 1,200 milligrams. Some doctors feel that just to be on the safe side, 1,500 milligrams should be consumed daily.

Here is a list of calcium rich foods:

CALCIUM COUNT

Food	Milligrams Calcium
1 cup skim milk	302
1 cup plain low-fat yogurt	452
1 large orange	54
1 cup beans	110
1 cup broccoli	135
1 cup spinach	167
1 cup kale	206
1 cup collard greens	220
1 cup mustard greens	284
6 ounces salmon	400

SODIUM

Sodium holds up to fifty times its own weight in water. Therefore most people are afraid to consume high-sodium foods because they will retain water. Excessive sodium consumption can in fact make you appear up to ten pounds heavier than you are, and can indeed cause your scale weight to rise by ten pounds. In addition, people with high blood pressure must avoid a high-sodium diet because it can aggravate the problem.

The RDA sets a maximum daily consumption of sodium at about 3,300 milligrams, while other health authorities suggest a maximum of 1,600 milligrams daily. Realistically speaking, if you keep your sodium between 1,500 and 2,500 milligrams daily—unless your doctor advises otherwise—you should be well within the healthy range, and you should not retain excessive water, especially if you drink plenty of water to flush out any excessive sodium in your digestive system.

Sodium is an essential mineral. Together with potassium it helps to regulate body fluids and maintain the acid–alkaline balance of the blood. Sodium is also responsible for muscle contraction; therefore a lack of it in the diet can cause severe cramping and even muscle shrinkage.

There is no lack of sodium in the American diet. Nearly everything we consume has some sodium in it—even tap water (10 milligrams in 8 ounces). Even an apple, a peach, or a potato has a trace of sodium. The following table describes the sodium content in several foods. (Note: vegetables are fresh or frozen.)

SODIUM CONTENT

Food (3½ ounces each)	Milligrams Sodium
Flounder	80
Sole	80
Beef	70
Chicken	60
Celery	25
Cabbage	20
Lettuce	4
Potatoes	3
Eggplant	2

High-Sodium Foods

So you see, even natural foods with no sodium added contain a fair amount of sodium. It's a good idea to avoid high-sodium foods such as canned foods, which can contain about 1,000 milligrams per cup, and frozen "diet" dinners, which also can contain about 1,000 milligrams of sodium per serving. Other high-sodium foods are anything that has been "smoked," foods containing MSG (Chinese food), and condiments such as mustard, ketchup, A-1 sauce, and Worchestershire sauce (500 to 1,000 milligrams per tablespoon).

There is never a need to add sodium to your food, yet people shake away at the table salt, pouring on at least 500 milligrams of sodium with each couple of shakes. (One commercial packet of salt contains 500 milligrams of sodium.)

Low-Fat, Low-Sodium Cooking with Spices, Vinegar, Wine, Lemon and Vegetable Juices

Learn to use spices—either alone or combined with vinegar and/or lemon or vegetable juice and/or wine—to replace sodium and high-fat cooking methods. Here is a list of spices and their compatible foods.

Allspice: fish, shellfish, sweet potatoes
Basil: fish, poultry, green vegetables, salads
Bay leaves: fish, stews
Cardamom: sweet potatoes
Chives: fish, baked potatoes, salads
Dill: fish, salad
Garlic powder: beef, chicken, fish, pork, pasta
Marjoram: poultry, green vegetables, salads
Oregano: chicken, eggplant, sauces
Rosemary: chicken
Sage: fish, poultry, soups, stews, stuffings
Tarragon: salmon, tomatoes, salad
Thyme: clams, fish, poultry, onions, squash
Turmeric: chicken, fish, pasta

You can be adventurous and sprinkle any combination of spices and juices into a tossed salad. You can cook things in combination with spices in regular white or red wine (*not* cooking wine, which is always high in sodium) or with fruit juices. (I cook fish and poultry in low-sodium tomato or V-8 juice.)

WATER

Water is the basis of all body fluids, including digestive juices, blood, urine, lymph, and perspiration. It is the primary carrier of nutrients throughout the body and is involved in nearly every body function, including absorption, digestion, excretion (if you are dehydrated, you may become constipated because it is water that keeps food moving through the intestinal tract), circulation, and lubrication. Body temperature is also regulated by water.

More than half the weight of the human body is water. We could live for a month or longer without food, but we would die in a few days without water.

Through perspiration and excretion, we use up and must replace about three quarts of water per day. Most fruits and vegetables are comprised of about 85 percent water, but such sources are not enough for water replacement. We must drink from six to eight 8-ounce glasses of liquid every day.

Can you count water-based drinks such as soups, juices, or coffee as your daily water requirement? Yes and no. While these liquids do replenish the body with moisture, they do not give the inner body the "shower" that pure water provides. In addition, caffeine has a diuretic effect, which increases water elimination, requiring you to ingest more water. Your best bet is to drink at least five 8-ounce glasses of clear water each day. A glass of water before each meal and one upon awakening and before bed will accomplish this goal.

Drinking lots of water helps to improve the complexion. It makes your skin appear younger and refreshed. If you start drinking lots of water, you will notice the change in your skin in a matter of days. Water also helps to curb the appetite, because many times when we think we are hungry, we are really just feeling dehydrated, and our poor body knows that we will not give it water, so it leads us to food to get its moisture.

Don't be concerned that if you drink lots of water you will retain water. The opposite is true. In fact, the more water you drink, the less you will retain, because water helps to flush water-retaining sodium from your system.

Types of Water

Water can be found in the tap and in other forms such as "natural," spring, purified, mineral, club soda, and seltzer. Natural water has not been modified by addition or deletion of minerals, while purified water (distilled or condensed water) is modified to remove minerals. Mineral water has been modified to add minerals. Club soda is carbonated water with added minerals, including sodium. Seltzer is carbonated water, sometimes with added minerals but without added sodium.

I drink plain old tap water sometimes, but lately, I've taken to drinking bottled spring water. It flows out of the earth on its own, is bottled near its source, and is unmodified by the addition or deletion of minerals. I like everything natural, and like to believe that I am drinking natural water, but if the truth be told, my joy may be purely psychological, because for all I know, the spring water I am drinking is bottled from somebody's tap in Brooklyn, New York!

CAFFEINE

I am able to drink two to three cups of regular drip caffeinated coffee daily without any problem. In some people, however, caffeine can cause heart irregularities, fibrocystic breast tissue, stress, decreased blood flow to the brain, nausea, insomnia, fast pulse, increased need to urinate, and raised cholesterol levels.

In addition, the caffeine habit can be difficult to break, although I found no problem dropping caffeine, just to see if I could do it. I had been drinking two to three cups of coffee daily for at least twenty years. I stopped cold and didn't start again for four months. I did not feel tired, but for the first three days I did get headaches. After that I was fine. Why did I start up again? Frankly, I just missed my cup of coffee. I am again back to my two to three cups a day, and until I have a problem, I will continue to enjoy them. You, on the other hand, must decide, with the advice of your doctor, what is right for you.

ALCOHOL

Some people are unable to handle any alcohol because they will overindulge or because they are alcoholics. Others can handle an occasional drink without a problem. I fall into the latter category and enjoy a few drinks on an occasional weekend evening.

Whether you enjoy a glass or two of wine with dinner as often as every evening or a drink or two on a weekend evening, moderate drinking will not hurt you; in fact, it may help you. Researchers at Harvard's School of Public Health did a study of men, ages forty to seventy-five, over a two-year period, and they discovered that those men who drank light to moderate amounts of alcohol (not more than one or two drinks a day) had a 25 to 40 percent lower chance of developing heart disease.

Keep in mind that the above discussion involves light to moderate drinking. Heavy drinking will *cause* rather than help prevent heart disease. If you don't drink at all now, should you start drinking in the hope that you will prevent heart disease? Of course not. Why add calories to your diet and force yourself to begin doing something that is indeed very controversial.

If you do drink, what should you drink in order to keep your calories low? Stick to white or red wine, champagne, or hard liquor with plain soda or fruit juices. Never indulge in mixed drinks that involve added sweeteners. Not only will this increase your calories, but it will increase your chance of getting sick and/or having a hangover. (Incidentally, I think two drinks a day are too much. Save your two drinks for one day a week. That would be much better for your diet too!)

BEVERAGE CHOICES

When trying to lose fat, the idea, as discussed above, is to create a calorie deficit. Keep your beverages to the nonfat area: seltzer, club soda, diet soda (this is your choice; some researchers are still in doubt as to the health hazards of diet soda), coffee, Postum or Pero (coffee substitutes), tea, and herbal tea. In general, it's not a good idea to drink fruit juices because they give you too much of an insulin boost and because it is better to eat the high-fiber, more-filling fruit.

BOTTOMS UP! EATING GUIDELINES

Now that you know all about good nutrition, it's time to put it all together in the following guidelines. (Please reread this chapter from time to time, until it becomes a part of your unconscious knowledge).

1. Eat 20 to 25 grams of fat per day. No more. If you do go over that amount, forgive yourself and resolve to do better the next day. Most people consume more than double the above amount, so if you slip once in a while, don't be too hard on yourself.

2. Eat a minimum of five times a day: three meals plus two snacks.

3. You may have three to five limited complex carbohydrate servings daily.

4. Eat two or three fruits a day. As a general rule, do not substitute fruit for juice. Don't eat fruit on an empty stomach, because you will get a quick energy burst and then an energy letdown.

5. Eat two to three protein choices per day.

6. Never go hungry. Eat unlimited complex carbohydrates anytime you are hungry. Carry those snacks around with you in plastic baggies.

7. To satisfy hunger and to prevent constant picking, eat complex carbohydrates that have low calorie-high density, such as potatoes, other vegetables, pasta, rice, and oatmeal.

8. If you are tempted to break your good eating habits and would like a treat, then instead of eating a fatty sweet such as a doughnut, indulge in two or three teaspoons of jam, seven hard candies, or one portion of a low- or nonfat sugary dessert, but keep these limited to three times per week.

9. You don't have to count calories, but be aware. Once in a while, calculate your daily calorie intake at the end of the day. You should be within the 1,500 to 2,000 range. Never go below 1,000 calories. That may slow down your metabolism to a "survival" state, and you may lose even less weight than you would have, had you kept your calories within the healthy weight-loss range.

10. Try to drink five 8-ounce glasses of clear water per day.

A WEEK OF DAILY MEAL PLANS

Here is a week of meal plans. For additional suggestions and interesting recipes, see bibliography under "Nutrition, Diet, and Cookbooks."

Note: You may enjoy any no-calorie beverage before, during, or after any meal, and anytime night or day. Beverages will not be mentioned in the following menus.

MONDAY

Breakfast

1 low-fat bran muffin
½ cup blueberries

Snack

whole-wheat pita bread with tofu and tomatoes and spices

Lunch

4 ounces tuna in water, mixed with chopped onions, cucumbers, and vinegar
2 slices whole wheat bread with lettuce and tomatoes and no-fat mayonnaise
tossed green salad

Snack

1 cup no-butter popcorn
pear

Dinner

6 ounces haddock
1 cup okra
1 cup collard greens
⅔ cup brown rice
tossed salad

Snack

1 cucumber
1 cup grapes

TUESDAY

Breakfast

bowl of whole-grain cold cereal with skim milk
15 cherries

Snack

⅔ cup cottage cheese
¼ honeydew melon

Lunch

bowl low-fat vegetable soup
1 cup Chinese cabbage
tossed salad
½ whole-grain bagel and 2 tablespoons jelly

Snack

1 sliced tomato and ½ head of lettuce
banana

Dinner

6 ounces sea bass
1 sweet potato
1 cup zucchini
1 cup rhubarb

Snack

1 apple
1 cup broccoli and cauliflower mix

WEDNESDAY

Breakfast

bowl of oatmeal
½ cantaloupe

Snack

2 large sliced cucumbers and 2 large sliced red peppers with vinegar and
  spices
bag of sliced carrots

Lunch

4 ounces tuna in water, mixed with vinegar and chopped cucumbers
2 slices whole wheat toast

Snack

lettuce and tomato salad
3 kumkwats

Dinner

6 ounces white-meat chicken
1 cup broccoli and cauliflower mix
1 cup summer squash
pasta shells and tomato sauce
large tossed salad

Snack

1 cup hot low-sodium broth
½ cup chopped celery

THURSDAY

Breakfast

1 poached egg and two egg whites
1 sliced tomato with vinegar and oregano

Snack

2 slices whole wheat toast and 2 teaspoons jelly
or
2 slices whole wheat toast and 2 tablespoons nonfat cottage cheese

Lunch

⅔ cup low-fat cottage cheese
1 large tossed salad
½ cup beets
1 cup spinach
½ grapefruit

Snack

1 ear of corn on the cob

Dinner

4 ounces (dry weight) whole wheat or artichoke pasta
4–8 ounces low-fat tomato sauce
1 cup cabbage
1 large tossed salad

Snack

bowl of oatmeal
1 cup raspberries

FRIDAY

Breakfast

whole-grain English muffin and 2 teaspoons jelly or ½ cup sliced strawberries
2 tangerines

Snack

two sliced red peppers with vinegar

Lunch

⅔ cup cottage cheese
large tossed salad
2 slices whole wheat toast

Snack

1 sliced cucumber
2 plums

Dinner

6 ounces pike
1 cup yellow beans
tossed salad
4 ounces pasta (dry weight)

Snack

baked potato
1 mango

SATURDAY

Breakfast

2 eggs scrambled with no fat
2 slices whole wheat toast

Snack

1 Chinese apple

Lunch

bowl of low-fat chicken-with-rice soup
4 low-fat whole-wheat crackers
large tossed salad
½ grapefruit

Snack

2 ounces pretzels

Dinner

6 ounces white-meat turkey
1 cup brussels sprouts
1 cup eggplant
large tossed salad
⅔ cup wild rice

Snack

1 cup kale
1 cup papaya

SUNDAY

Breakfast

bowl of shredded wheat cereal with skim milk
3 fresh prunes

Snack

½ cup kidney beans in large bowl of escarole, mixed with radishes and
tomatoes

Lunch

½ whole wheat bagel with ¾ cup nonfat cottage cheese
large tossed salad
large slice watermelon

Snack

⅔ cup brown rice with diced tomatoes and chopped onion

Dinner

6 ounces flounder
1 cup spinach
1 cup mixed vegetables
large tossed salad

Snack

1 cup green beans
1 large peach

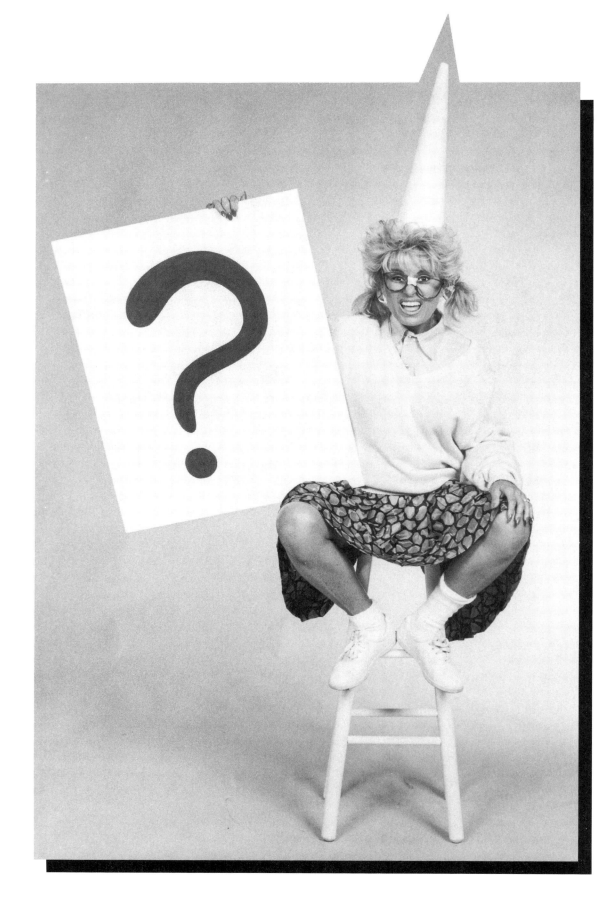

10

IT'S NOT A STUPID QUESTION

Now that you've read the book, you're ready to get started. But just when you're about to begin your workout, or shortly after you do, a question comes to mind. Did I cover it in the book? Perhaps I did, but you certainly can't find it. You look in the index, under all possible alphabetical designations. You still can't find it. You want to write to me, but you really wish you could have the answer NOW. Well, chances are, you can because you will probably find that your question and answer are found in the following pages.

Here are the forty-one questions most commonly asked by people who write to me saying, "I know this is probably a stupid question, but..." Well, the fact is it's not a stupid question. In fact, your question is probably one that many other women thought of, too!

If after reading this chapter, you discover that I have still not answered your question, or if you want to contact me for any other reason, please write to me at my P.O. box, provided at the end of this chapter. Be sure to include a stamped, self-addressed envelope if you wish a reply.

1. I want to start working with weights and developing those feminine muscles all over my body, but I heard that if you get muscles, they will turn to fat if you ever stop working out. If this is true, I'm not going to work out because—who knows?—I may decide at some point I don't want to do this program anymore.

This is one of the most common myths floating around in the fitness world. Let me assure you once and for all, with the entire world of medical authority behind me, muscle can never turn to fat. It never has, and it never will. Muscle and fat cells are completely different, structurally and functionally. When you build muscle, you actually lose fat, for two reasons:

1. You use up calories in the workout itself (about 265 per session with Bottoms Up!, for example)

2. You increase the rate at which your body burns calories (your metabolic rate increases), because muscle is always using energy even while you are sleeping or sitting in a chair.

But what happens if you stop working out? Simply put, your muscles slowly shrink until they return to where they were before you started working out.

2. I've always had a problem with cellulite, and believe it or not, my boyfriend has some cellulite, too. What is cellulite anyway? Can we get rid of it by dieting and working out? Can a man do the Bottoms Up! Workout?

Cellulite is bunched-up fat; in other words, it is "dimpled" fat. You don't see cellulite on men as much as on women because men tend to hold most of their excess fat in the abdominal area, where fat generally forms into a smooth roll rather than bunched-up layers. Women tend to store fat in three places: the stomach, the thighs, and the hips/buttocks. Fat tends to bunch up when it is stored on the thighs and hips/buttocks, so overweight women usually have more of a cellulite problem than overweight men. In addition, women generally have thinner skin than men, and carry more fat cells.

Both men and women will get rid of all cellulite as they follow this workout and low-fat eating plan. You can tell your boyfriend to start out by doing the Gut Busters Workout (my abdominal program that is addressed to men who claim they just want to get rid of their gut; by the way, women can do it, too), and then have him join you in Bottoms Up! for a total-body workout. If he does decide to do Bottoms Up!, let him know that he can skip the hip/buttock exercises, because men do not store fat in this area. He will get more than enough hip/buttock exercises just by doing his thigh routine (these exercises also help to shape the buttocks).

3. I have chronic neck and back pain. I've tried every doctor you could imagine, and they can't seem to find the problem or do anything for me. My best friend says she used to have the same problem, and her doctor referred her to a chiropractor. I was surprised, because I didn't know that chiropractors can really help. I thought they were just quacks. What do you think?

First of all, much lower back pain is caused by weak abdominal muscles, because it is the abdominal muscles that support the back. After a few months of doing the abdominal workout in this book, chances are you will experience less and less back pain. But what if you still have neck pain, and perhaps even some lingering back pain? It could be due to tension in your daily life or misalignments of various kinds.

Chiropractors can indeed help. In fact, I see one myself for an occasional stiff neck. Chiropractors find and correct vertebral subluxations (vertebrae twisted out of normal alignment through excessive stress of various kinds). They do this by adjusting the bones back into alignment. This releases the pressure on the nerves and not only alleviates back and neck pain but helps improve overall health.

Total-body exercise, such as the workout described in this book, and chiropractic work hand in hand to help keep the muscles that support the frame strong. Chiropractic helps athletes and people working out, engaging in a sport, or even just performing daily functions such as walking and sitting to operate at their peak levels of performance without pain. In summary, I highly recommend that you pay a visit to your local chiropractor. You may be pleasantly surprised with the results. You can find a good chiropractor in your area by calling The International Chiropractic Association at 703-528-5000.

4. I was desperate to lose ten pounds for a wedding that was only a month away, and I went on a liquid diet for four weeks. I lost ten pounds and fit into my dress, but right after the wedding, I couldn't stop myself from eating, and now, a month later, I have gained it all back, with five more pounds in the bargain. Can liquid diets work, or are they all doomed to fail?

Liquid diets, which were originally developed for very obese people who were in life-and-death trouble, are not meant for most of us. In fact, they are an unnatural way to eat—even if you do allow yourself one solid meal a day. The human body was built to eat a well-balanced diet of chewable food. That's why, after the first year of life (usually sooner), babies are weaned from a liquid diet of milk and put on solid foods.

If we deny the body the opportunity to chew and ingest solid food, we create a "deprivation" sense in our unconscious minds, and the moment we are off the liquid diet, we eat and eat and eat. Coming off the diet, we feel as if it is a life-and-death situation, and instead of having the discipline to go for the healthy, low-fat foods, we eat anything in sight, in response to an unconscious fear that solid food will soon become unavailable again.

In addition, liquid diets often force you to keep your calories so low that you border on the starvation level. The combination of the two—the lack of a substantial amount of solid food (the chewing experience) and lack of life-sustaining calories—trigger the "starvation response" the moment you are off guard. In your case, once the wedding was over, you let down your guard and began eating to make up for lost time, and quite naturally you gained back what you lost, with some extra pounds in the bargain.

The fact is that the only way to lose weight is to do it slowly and with a well-balanced diet of chewable foods that make you feel full and satisfied.

5. I am anxious to lose weight, and although I'm following your low-fat eating plan and the weight is coming off a pound or two a week, I'm impatient and want to lose faster. Should I take diet pills or fat-burning enzymes to speed things up a bit?

When it comes to losing permanent weight, there are no shortcuts. Diet pills, which are composed of heavy doses of caffeine or other drugs, accelerate your metabolism, making you burn more calories per hour. You do lose weight while you're taking the pills, but you can't take them forever (they eventually cause heart palpitations and other health problems), and when you stop taking them, your metabolism will have a regressive reaction. It will slow down—not to its previous "normal" speed, but even further, causing you to burn calories at a much slower rate than ever before in your life. This slowdown may last for months, causing you to gain weight eating the same amount of calories you previously ate to maintain your weight or even to lose weight. So my advice to you is don't be tempted into the temporary promise of diet pills. In the end they make your weight problem worse!

As far as "fat-burning enzymes" taken by bodybuilders, there is no proof whatsoever that these work to help you to burn fat. Frankly, I would stay away from all pills that claim to help you lose weight, and stick to well-balanced, low-fat nutritious eating. As the saying goes, "You can't fool Mother Nature."

6. I'm confused. I notice that in *Gut Busters*, you tell people that they can work just one body part, their stomach, and get results. I thought it was impossible to spot-reduce.

You were right in thinking it's impossible to spot-reduce—but it *is* possible to "spot-change." By doing the seven exercises in *Gut Busters* for fifteen minutes six days a week, you bomb away at your stomach with such intensity that you develop a steel girdle of muscle in the abdominal area. However, if a person is overweight, he or she must also follow the low-fat eating plan in the book, or the steel girdle of muscle will remain hidden under a layer of fat.

It is especially important to lose excess fat if you want muscles to show up in the stomach area, because the stomach is a favorite storage bin for fat—much more so than the arms, for example. In fact, if you wanted to spot-change your biceps, you could do that without even dieting. You could exercise only your biceps and develop a significant muscle there. Fat would not hide that muscle because the biceps is not a favorite storage place for fat.

The men and women who have used *Gut Busters* have proven once and for all that if you want to, you can indeed spot-change. Many of them have sent me their before and after photographs, showing me "washboard" or "beer-can" (not "beer-belly") stomachs, and some of these folks still have shapeless arms, legs, backs, and so on. If they want to get the rest of their bodies in shape, they will of course have to do a total-body workout.

In summary, it is not possible to spot-reduce by dieting, but it is possible to spot-change by working out the right way. When you come to think of it, that's exactly what you're doing with the Bottom's Up! Workout. You're spot-changing specific muscle groups as you exercise them with a carefully designed program. It is only because you choose to exercise all nine body parts that you get the result of a completely toned body.

7. I'm really confused. I went to this "abs" class at a health spa, and we worked our abs for a half-hour—nonstop. Is this the right way to work out?

No. Abs classes typically overtrain your abdominal muscles, so that you wear down muscle as you're building it. It's like taking one step forward and one step back. Let me prove it by my own example.

Before I knew what I was doing, I used to do five hundred sit-ups and leg raises every day, and yet I still had a slight pot on my lower stomach, and no definition whatsoever. Finally I ran into a bodybuilder in a gym who had what we call "washboard" abs. He saw me overtraining my stomach, and he tried to explain to me that I should work in sets of a variety of specific exercises—and that I shouldn't do more than fifteen to twenty-five repetitions per set. Afraid that if I did less I would look even worse than I already looked, I started to argue with him. Then suddenly I looked at his stomach, and I started to laugh at myself.

How foolish of me, I thought. *The man is telling you how to exercise your stomach—and you are arguing with him. Look at his stomach and look at yours, and then ask yourself if you should listen to him.*

I decided to follow his routine, and in a few months I had lost my pot and had beautiful definition in my entire abdominal area. Since then, I have learned a variety of stomach routines—all of them used by champion bodybuilders—and they are found in my various books.

Ironically, I was recently visiting a popular health resort and doing the abdominal routine contained in this book. The woman who runs the abdominal class came into the gym and noticed me working out, and she came over to correct me and to tell me that I should join her abdominal class instead of wasting my time doing what I was doing. I had a bulky sweatshirt on at the time, but when I noticed that her stomach was smooth and slightly protruding in the lower area, I couldn't resist lifting my shirt and pulling down my sweat pants just enough to show her my entire rippled, rock-hard, flat stomach. She stood there with her mouth open, then said, "Oh. You're a bodybuilder." I said, "No. Not at all. I just use the same techniques." She then asked me to show her my full routine.

8. My breasts are hanging practically to my waist. Can I really lift them by working out? Can I also make them bigger. I hope I won't lose my breasts like these female bodybuilders you see. Please tell me what to expect.

You can lift your breasts to some extent by developing muscles under them, and you can also make them appear larger, because the supporting pectoral muscles will help to create the look of cleavage. But working out with weights cannot actually increase the size of the breast itself, because the breast is made of fatty tissue. This is where males and females differ. We both have pectoral muscles in the chest area, but women have fatty tissue (breasts) above the pectoral muscle.

This brings me to the last part of your question. What about some of those female bodybuilders you see who seem to have lost their breasts completely? Have no fear. These women diet to the point where their body-fat level is often below 10 percent. When body-fat levels reach an extremely low level, the body is forced to give up its last bit of fat—even the healthy and desirable fatty tissue of the breast. In addition, these women use extremely heavy weights for their chest routine, hundreds of pounds, and they work much longer and harder on the chest. Although there is no scientific proof that such heavy training of the breast wears away fatty breast tissue, it seems obvious to me that it contributes to the problem.

In summary, in order to lose your breasts, you would have to diet and exercise like a bodybuilder—a diet and exercise program that is certainly *not* found in this book!

9. I notice that you recommend that we use the same weights for all body parts, and yet I find that I can go heavier on my chest, for example, than I can on my shoulders, and heavier on my biceps than I can on my triceps. Should I buy heavier dumbbells for these areas?

In the beginning, to keep things simple, you should use the same relatively light weights for all suggested body parts, unless you are a seasoned weight-trainer. Later, as you become familiar with the routine and your own body begins to tell you to go heavier on certain parts, you can use heavier weights for certain body parts. For example, I recommend three-, five-, and eight-pound dumbbells for all body parts to start out. (You may have to go even lighter than that in the beginning.) After you've been exercising for a few months, you will find that chest, biceps, back, calves, and thighs seem to demand heavier weights. When this happens, you will want to purchase a set or two of heavier dumbbells to accommodate them—say, tens, twelves, and perhaps later, fifteens or even twenties.

The bottom line is, the weight guide is general, but as you get used to the routine, you will instinctively know where to put in heavier weights and where to keep the weights lighter.

10. I am very upset. I've been following your workout for six weeks, and I went down two pants sizes, but when I got on the scale, I saw that I lost only seven and a half pounds. Then I started weighing myself every day, and the scale either stays the same or goes up a pound. I'm a size 7 and I look good, but I had set my mind to lose another seven pounds. What should I do?

You may not have to lose as much weight as you thought you had to lose. Another woman recently wrote to me saying that she wanted to lose fifty pounds. She followed the workout and diet for four months, saying that she didn't weigh herself because she knows muscle weighs more than fat and she didn't want to get discouraged. But she finally couldn't stand the mystery and got on the scale.

"Wow. Was I depressed," she said. "I only lost 22 pounds in four months. I know I'm smaller than 22 pounds weight loss. I'm wearing clothes I could wear only if I lost 35 pounds. I was shocked. I still have 28 pounds to lose."

The truth is, the woman does not have another twenty-eight pounds to lose now that her body composition has changed. In fact, she may only have to lose another eighteen pounds. Why? She now looks thinner at a higher weight. This happens to everyone who works with one of my programs.

I'll use myself as an example. Look at the "before" photograph of me at 115 pounds on page 11. I weighed the same, yet don't I look thinner now?

Muscle weighs more than fat but it takes up less space. As you are working with the weights, you are losing lots of lightweight fat, and at the same time you are adding gorgeous, tight, toned muscle that weighs *more* than fat. So forget the scale and start looking in the mirror. It's a reeducation, but once you rethink the meaning of *weight*, you'll finally realize that it's not what the scale says but what you see in the mirror that counts.

11. Since you say we should forget about the scale, does that mean we should never weigh ourselves? What about body-fat composition tests?

Of course I can't tell you to never again weigh yourself. In fact, I weigh myself from time to time—out of curiosity. My main point in deemphasizing the scale is this: now that you are working with weights and forming muscle that weighs more than fat but takes up less space, your weight will mean something different than it did before. You will look slimmer and be in shape (a smaller size, and tight and toned) at a higher weight than before. As long as you realize this (and also that water-weight fluctuates), the scale will no longer have a hold over you, and occasionally weighing yourself out of curiosity will not be a problem.

As far as tests measuring body fat, don't waste your time. They are another way to fill up your life with a lot of numbers that are not the true measure of your fitness. My body-fat level has been measured anywhere between 18 percent and 23 percent—and look at me. If I were going to concern myself with body-fat measures, I would diet myself down like a near-anorexic. I look in the mirror, and if I look good, that's all I care about.

The funny thing about body-fat measure scales is that some people can have a very low measure and still be out of shape. I took the test next to a badly out of shape, thin but flabby woman who measured in at 18 percent! She looked at me and bragged, "My body fat is only 17 percent. What's yours?" When I told her it was 23 percent, she walked away with a smug expression. "How silly," I thought. "Does she ever look in the mirror?" In my view that woman was a perfect example of a soft, flabby "skinny-fat." She may not have much fat on her body, but she didn't have much muscle tone either.

12. I used to think working out to get in shape was just for those who are overly concerned with the outward appearance. Now I realize that preoccupation with my weight is a bigger drain on my happiness than any other factor in my life. Will this workout make me feel better about myself—even if my main goal is not to show off my body?

Yes. This workout will make you feel better about yourself in every way, even if you never intend to show off your body to another living soul. We've all heard the expression "Sound body, sound mind." When your body is tight and toned, there is a subtle transference to your mind—a message to your unconscious that says, "You are in control."

In addition, because of the reality of dealing with a very fitness-oriented society, when we are not overweight and/or out of shape, the world looks at us with a more positive eye, and we are not forced to continually ward off negative feedback and are no longer tempted to explain or apologize for the state of our bodies. In short, we are free to put our energy into achieving our goals in life.

13. You look so healthy. Which vitamins and supplements do you take? I want to try them.

I do not take any vitamins, although I have tried them. Somehow, after a day or two, I can't bring myself to put them in my mouth. Something seems to be telling me that they will throw my system off, so I just stick to plain old food.

Interestingly, I followed the same system with my daughter once she was ten years old, with the blessing of her pediatrician. He said that if you eat a well-balanced diet, you don't need vitamins or food supplements.

I believe that taking vitamins can trick your body into believing that you are eating a balanced diet when you are not, and that you may pass on foods you would ordinarily crave, because the vitamins will make you think that you don't need them. Let me give you an example. From time to time, for reasons unknown to me, I will be passing the bananas or the liver or the kidney beans in the supermarket, and I will be compelled to buy these items. I don't like the taste of them, but I suddenly get a craving for them—so I buy them, and I eat them with relish. Why do I do this? I believe that my body is telling me that I need the vitamins contained in these foods.

If I took vitamins just as a backup, I feel that I might not have these urges, and I might miss out on the real food that all doctors agree is always better than vitamins or supplements.

However, I don't want to go on record as saying I don't believe in vitamins or supplements, because I do believe that they can be helpful for many people. I just feel that way for myself at this point. Who knows? At some future date I may change my mind and begin taking vitamins and supplements myself. In any case, you should speak to your doctor and/or nutritionist, and then decide for yourself what is best for you.

14. My thighs are very big. How can I trim them down with extra work, besides working with weights?

To trim down extra-big thighs, the best exercise is the stationary bike, set at the lowest tension as you move your legs as quickly as possible. If you do this exercise for thirty minutes four to six times a week, you will notice a marked reduction in your thigh size in six to twelve weeks, and what's more, you'll be burning extra fat because bike riding is a straight aerobic activity.

15. Can you recommend exercises to lose weight in or tighten up the face and neck?

I get this question a lot, and I always hate answering it because the answer is not what people want to hear. The fact is, there is no exercise that will remove wrinkles from the face and neck. As you know from reading this book, exercising puts definition and muscle on various body parts. The last thing you want is definition on your face and neck (lines that would look like wrinkles) or muscles (which would make your face and neck look fatter).

I know that there are facial exercise programs around, but I don't believe they work. At best, they are a waste of time, and at worst, they make the problem worse. What is the answer? Either grow old gracefully or pay a visit to the cosmetic surgeon. I intend to do a little bit of both!

16. Can I do this workout if I'm pregnant?

You can do this workout, with your doctor's permission, through your fifth or sixth month. Then, again with your doctor's permission, switch to the 12-Minute Total-Body Workout, in addition to walking 30 to 45 minutes a day through your eighth or ninth month. Once the baby is born, you can do the 12-Minute Total-Body Workout for two to three weeks, then go right back to this workout—again, all of this with your doctor's permission.

17. I'm a vegetarian. How can I adapt your diet to my needs?

I suggest that you consume one-half your body weight in protein grams. If you weigh 120 pounds, this means you will consume about 60 grams of protein a day, but you can consume as low as 44 grams per day if you so choose. You can follow a vegetarian diet by substituting vegetable sources of protein for animal protein. There are 10 grams of protein in a cup of beans, 8 grams in a cup of skim milk, and 17 grams in a cup of yogurt. Other sources of nonanimal protein are tofu and egg whites. For other vegetarian suggestions, see the bibliography in my book *Supercut: Nutrition for the Ultimate Physique.*

18. Should I start the workout before I lose the weight? I'm worried that I'm big enough already with all of my fat—I don't want to get even bigger.

One of the worst mistakes you could make would be to wait until you reach your weight goal before beginning the workout. Why? Because working out will help you to lose the weight by burning additional fat and by creating muscle that in and of itself burns fat twenty-four hours a day. Don't worry that the muscle you are building will expand your body outward and make you look even fatter than you do now. In fact, the muscle that you are building will be small and condensed and will take up less space than the fat you are losing. What's more, once you lose the fat, your tight, toned body will be waiting for you, rather than the loose, flabby, "skinny-fat" body that would be waiting for you if you didn't work out *while* you were losing the weight.

19. How can I get bigger muscles in my calves or thighs?

The same principle holds true for gaining size in these body parts as does for gaining size in any body part: you must use heavier weights and rest longer between sets, about forty-five to sixty seconds. If you wish to gain significant muscle size, you can follow the size-gaining plans found on pages 81 and 222–223, or you can get a copy of my book *Now or Never*, which specifically deals with building more size (see page 286).

20. I have a flat exercise bench, and it's too much trouble to put books under the foot of the bench to make it go to an incline. What will happen if I do the incline exercises with the bench flat?

If you do this, it will mean doubling up on the flat exercises. You will miss out on the varied angle that the incline position allows, but you will still see excellent results in your workout. You will simply lose a little of the balance of the workout.

21. My thighs are really out of shape. Will they be perfect in three months, or will they lag behind my other body parts? What about my horrible stomach and buttocks? In other words, do different body parts take longer on some people?

Most people have a "troublesome" body part or two, areas that take longer than others to shape up. For most women these body parts are the thighs, the hips/buttocks, and the stomach. Since *Bottoms Up!* puts the emphasis on exactly these body parts, bombing them with the maximum of exercise, you should see results sooner than you did with any other workout, and many of you will have achieved your goal in a few months. However, depending upon your particular genetic makeup and the extent to which your muscles have been neglected, these body parts may take as long as a year to perfect.

Please don't become disgusted. So what if it takes you a year to have gorgeous, sexy thighs where you used to have "cheesecake" cellulite-ridden thighs? So what if it takes a year to lift dimply, droopy buttocks and make them high, round, and firm. So what if it takes a full year to remove your potbelly and net you a flat, defined, rock-hard stomach? It would be worth the work even if it took two years, because once you get it, it is yours for life—and once you have it, it doesn't take nearly as much work to maintain it.

22. I'm sixty-eight years old, and frankly, at my age I couldn't care less about reshaping my body. Nobody ever sees it, and I like it that way. I'm not overweight, I do aerobics and have a strong heart and lungs, but I am weak, and I'd like to do some strength training. Is your workout for me?

This workout is perfect for you, even if you could care less about your appearance, because it will strengthen your overall body musculature and increase your overall bone density. Medical research has now proven that people build bone and muscle at any age—even in their nineties.

You are smart to want to gain strength at this point in your life, because this will serve as an insurance policy for a quality life as you approach your golden years. After all, even the healthiest heart and lungs won't pick you up off the floor if your muscles and bones are too weak to assist you!

You should do this workout just like everybody else, breaking in gently and then going full-force into the program.

23. I know you've written three books besides *Bottoms Up!* Which book is best for my purposes?

Now or Never, my first weight-training book, helps you to build slightly bigger muscles than you will build with this workout. *The Fat Burning Workout* will net you slightly smaller muscles than this workout. *The 12-Minute Total-Body Workout* will net you the smallest muscles of all the workouts. Most people will want to switch back and forth, doing all four workouts for three months to a year at a time to prevent boredom, and to net the perfectly seasoned body. See page 221–223 for more details on these workouts.

24. I'm following the Weight Watchers diet, and my husband is following the Pritikin diet. Can we follow these diets and do your workout, or do we have to follow your diet exactly?

Both of those diets are excellent, well-balanced diets that are low in fat and high in carbohydrates. You will notice that both of these diets suggest a little less protein than I do, and the Pritikin diet requires a little less fat (10 percent). This is fine. Lower fat and lower protein will not hinder your progress. As long as you keep your complex carbohydrates high (for energy) and your fat low, you will lose maximum fat and make progress in your shape-up plan.

I suggest slightly higher protein than do these diets because it is my experience that bodies that work with weights and are building muscle require more protein than bodies that do not work with weights. Perhaps this is because muscles themselves are made of protein. Chances are you will notice yourself wanting to eat slightly more protein than you did in the past once you have been working out with this program for a few weeks. If you don't, or if your doctor or alternate diet indicates you shouldn't, there is no problem.

25. If I lose weight, will my skin sag?

If you lose a significant amount of weight and you do not work out with weights as suggested in this or one of my other workout books, your skin is likely to sag. If you follow this program, however, you will be building firm muscles under your skin. As you lose the weight, instead of sagging, your skin will adapt itself, surrounding and clinging to the shapely muscles as they form.

26. I can't do sit-ups, leg raises, squats, or lunges. Are there substitute exercises for these movements?

Yes. Just follow the exercise instructions for the "therapeutic alternative" for each exercise that you cannot do. I have provided substitutes for all the exercises that might prove difficult for those who have back or knee problems. This is a first for me, and long overdue.

27. Joyce, not too long ago, I saw you on a talk show discussing a book you wrote called *Get Rid of Him*. How does *Get Rid of Him* fit into your workout business, or does it?

As you may know, fitness is not my only concern. My Ph.D. is in English literature, with a specialization in psychology and for years I have been writing inspirational books for parents and teens. *Get Rid of Him*, however, is probably the most important book I've ever written. It is addressed to women, both single and married, who find themselves in relationships that drain their energy and that are more trouble than they're worth, and it inspires women to leave such relationships, while teaching them how to build self-esteem.

And in fact, *Get Rid of Him is* linked to fitness. You see, if a woman is out of shape, she may allow whatever negative feelings she has about her body to affect her self-esteem. When this happens, she may convince herself to stay with a man, even if he isn't good for her, falsely believing that if she leaves him, she will never find another man.

Get Rid of Him inspires women to leave a man, no matter what, and then it helps women to do whatever they have to do to feel better about themselves—and getting in shape is often one of those things.

28. How fast am I allowed to go when I am doing the exercises? What if I want to slow down, or even take a rest when I'm not supposed to. For example, what if I break up a twin set and rest between a chest and shoulder exercise?

If you use relatively light weights, you will be able to go quite fast. If you use heavier weights, you will naturally move a little slower. If you take rests even between the exercises of the twin sets, you will still get full muscle shaping, but you will lose a little of the fat-burning effect, and of course, you will lose time. If you find yourself wanting to rest even between the exercises of an interset, you might want to lower your overall weight load and wait until you are stronger to add the weight again.

29. You say "feel the flex in your muscles." How can I feel my muscles flex?

The way I teach someone to flex a muscle is by using an imaginary attack as an example: Make believe I am coming at you full force, ready to punch you in the stomach with all of my might. What do you do? You tighten your stomach in preparation for the attack. This hardening, defensive movement of your stomach muscles is called flexing your stomach.

Try this method with your arm. Put your arm straight down at your side and make believe I am a doctor, coming at your upper arm with a long, sharp needle, about to give you an injection. What do you do? Perhaps you close your eyes or look away, but you definitely flex (squeeze) your upper arm muscle (biceps and triceps) in defense.

If you want to flex a muscle, just imagine something coming at that muscle to attack it, and imagine your natural defense, a squeezing together movement of the muscle fibers.

30. I was always a poor dieter, but with this plan I have lost seventy pounds, and yet I eat so much food. People don't understand how I can eat so much and still lose weight. Can you help me to explain this to them.

I invented this diet because I am the worst dieter in the world. If I can't have food when and where I want it, I feel deprived and resentful—and in fact, I rebel and end up eating junk food. But since I learned how to eat the right way, and discovered that it's not how much you eat but what you eat, I eat loads of unlimited complex carbohydrates anytime, night or day, like you. This, coupled with the allowed fruits, low-fat protein, and limited complex carbohydrates such as potatoes, pasta, and bagels, makes it seem like I always have something in my mouth.

Your friends can't believe that you can eat so much and yet lose weight, because in the past they probably saw you eat less—but of the wrong foods. For example, before, you may have eaten only four ounces of potato chips, but those chips contained 30 grams of fat. Now you're probably eating loads of vegetables, a couple of fruits, and even a couple of slices of bread. All of them combined have about three grams of fat.

31. Can I eat before bedtime?

Good news. Yes, you can. Recent research indicates that it doesn't much matter when you eat. What's more important is to eat often (don't starve yourself all day and eat one huge meal at the end of the day) and to keep your fat low. The only problem with eating just before bedtime is, you may not be able to sleep soundly because your digestive system will still be processing the food.

I must admit that this never bothered me. In fact, I always snack all evening if I'm home, right up until bedtime, and if I'm out for the evening, I make myself quite a spread of unlimited complex carbohydrates—and even a slice or two of whole wheat bread—just before bedtime.

32. I notice that in your previous books you left out all inner-thigh work. Why do you suddenly give so many inner thigh exercises now?

In my previous books I left out all inner-thigh work because up until that point the exercises I had tried put a thick muscle in that area that looked like fat. The regular thigh exercises shaped the thigh so beautifully, and the inner thigh seemed to fall naturally into place—without a muscle. (See my photographs in *The Fat-Burning Workout*, for example.)

However, so many women were writing to me, asking for special exercises for the inner thigh that I was driven to do further research, and I came up with a series of inner thigh exercises for *Bottoms Up!* that give inner thigh tone and definition without the bulk. In fact, if you look closely, you will see that my inner thigh is more defined and that my legs look better than ever before. So my improved leg workout is due to you, my wonderful readers.

33. I often feel weak and need energy. What can I eat that won't make me fat but will give me an energy boost that will last a while?

The good old baked or boiled potato is your answer. It is high in density and low in calories (see page 242) and fills you up, but what's more, it is composed of complex carbohydrates that provide gradually released energy for hours after eating. If you're really hungry, eat two potatoes. You can spice them up with mustard, salsa, or nonfat yogurt, or eat them plain. In any case, the stomach holds only two to three pounds of food, so two large baked potatoes will definitely take away that empty feeling of deprivation.

34. What is the best way to get rid of stretch marks?

Stretch marks occur when connective tissue is stretched beyond its capacity. This sometimes happens after pregnancy, or after a person has lost a great deal of weight that had been carried for a very long time.

Retin-A has been known to completely remove almost all traces of stretch marks when taken under a doctor's guidance, but it is not known whether or not these marks will return. Retin-A can produce troublesome side effects, such as peeling, swelling, and redness of skin. Also, because it is possible that Retin-A can cause birth defects, doctors will not prescribe it for women who are planning to have children, who are pregnant, or even who are nursing.

Incidentally, Retin-A is not officially approved by the FDA for treating stretch marks or wrinkles. It is only approved for treating acne.

More-traditional remedies, such as stretch creams, can temporarily hide stretch marks, but the moment you stop using the cream, the marks become as visible as they were before.

On the up side, if you follow this workout, your body will be so completely reshaped and defined that your new musculature and definition will greatly help to take the focus of attention away from any stretch marks that you may have.

35. Joyce, tell us the truth. What do you really do? I mean, exactly what workout do you follow to look the way you do?

I do what I tell you to do in the maintenance section of this book. I switch back and forth among the plans in my books, *Bottoms Up!, The Fat-Burning Workout, Now or Never, The 12-Minute Total-Body Workout,* and from time to time I include *Gut Busters* in my routine. My present figure is the result of learning as I go along. Now I am doing the Bottoms Up! Workout, with the Wild Woman Workout for arms and the Terminator Workout for chest, shoulders, and back. I work out four or five days a week, but when I'm trying to look my best, I work out six days a week.

As far as aerobics go, I either walk for forty minutes or run for twenty to twenty-five minutes six days a week. I do this because I love to eat, and the extra aerobics allow me that much more play. Once in a while, when I really get in trouble—say, when I've started to pig out not only on my one day a week but three or four days a week, and the pounds slowly get on me, and I've got to get them off for a television show or a photo shoot—I'll do all of the above and add in an extra thirty-minute bike-riding session five or six days a week.

That program is hell—but I do it because in an emergency it works. My biggest problem is fitting the workout into my busy schedule—and getting my sometimes lazy body to do it. But by an act of will, I do it, because I know the results are guaranteed.

And by the way, once those pounds get on me, they come off very, very slowly, because I don't have a lot to lose, and as mentioned before, the body likes a few extra pounds in case of a future famine. Sometimes I lose nothing for three weeks, even though I've been dieting and exercising like mad. Then suddenly the scale will drop two or three pounds. Then I can go another month as the scale goes up and down a pound, and finally another two pounds will drop off.

Am I contradicting myself by weighing myself when I tell you not to do it? No. I weigh myself only so that I can have a true story to tell you and so that I can comfort you about the treacherous scale—and to encourage you not to base your progress on it. The fact is, I rarely weigh myself unless I'm doing it to prove a point in my books. I use the mirror as my guide.

36. I have been following your workout faithfully six days a week for three months, and I've seen amazing results. But once in a while, something comes up, and I don't get to work out for three or four days at a time. I look in the mirror and I think that I have lost it all. Is this my imagination? How fast do you lose what you've gotten if you stop working out?

Don't worry. If you stop working out for a few days or even for a week or more, you don't lose everything you've worked for. In fact, it takes as long to lose what you have as it took you to get it. Let me explain. If you worked out for a year, it would take a year of not working out to lose the muscle tone you had gained.

But there's great news. It would take you only one-third the time to get back that muscle tone once you started working out again, because muscles "remember." For example, if you stopped working out, even for a year, and then started working out again, it would take you only about four months to get back to the conditioning that it previously took a year to achieve. Once you start working out, it's like having muscles in the bank.

37. I was a bodybuilder and I have big muscles. I want to do your program for a while. Will I lose my muscles?

If you were used to working with much heavier weights and taking long rests between sets, your muscle size will eventually go down a bit if you follow this program—but not by very much. The Bottoms Up! Workout is designed to give maximum hardness and definition, while at the same time allowing for significant muscle development. If you already have large muscles, this workout will certainly maintain them—at least to 75 percent. If you do lose some size, you can always switch to the Now or Never Workout, and in a matter of months you can get it back.

38. You mention that as we get stronger and stronger, over time we should raise our weights. We are starting out with threes, fives, and eights. How long does it usually take to get strong enough to raise the weights? Another thing—just how high in weight will I eventually go? I mean, will I eventually be using hundred-pound weights?

Good question. Everyone is different. Some people find themselves strong enough to raise their overall weights in a matter of three weeks or less, while others take as long as two or three months. The most important thing to remember about raising the weights is to do it when the work has become too easy and you know that you are not working to capacity. Remember, the harder you work, the better will be your result.

Of course you will never be using hundred-pound dumbbells. You will reach a "plateau" and stay there. I use tens, fifteens, and twenties, but it took me over a year to reach this point. To be honest, I do go a little slower for my last set than for my first two and, in fact, sometimes even rest a few seconds where I shouldn't rest. But I want to use the heavier weights because I like having slightly larger muscles.

39. My two best friends and I are in an argument. One friend claims that you can get your thighs, hips, and butt in shape with step aerobics. The other says the stair-stepping machine will do it. I say you can't get your thighs, hips, and butt in shape with either method, and that you have to use a workout like the ones found in your books. What argument can I give to prove my point?

The only thing step aerobics and stair stepping machines can do for these areas is to strengthen them and to help to build overall endurance, while at the same time burning some fat. In order to sculpt and reshape the thigh and hip/buttock area, you must work out in carefully designed sets of specific exercises, done in a specified sequence—the way bodybuilders do, only with lighter weights. In working with the weights, you sculpt and shape the muscle the way an artist would sculpt and shape with clay. Stepping and benching simply cannot sculpt.

40. Is it really true that once you reach your weight goal—or I should say, your ideal shape—you can eat anything you want all day once a week? I don't see how you could get away with this and not get fat?

It certainly is true, and here's why. You will be eating a low-fat diet all week (20 to 25 grams of fat) and keeping your calories below 2,000, and you will be doing the Bottoms Up! Workout. If you did not have a "pig-out" day once a week, you would continue to lose weight—over time. Of course that weight loss would be slow, because when the body is at its ideal weight, it resists weight loss. Nevertheless, in a matter of months you would lose more weight. By eating whatever you want one day a week, the body balances itself out and makes up for the low-fat diet during the week. You end up maintaining your weight.

This system works. I've been advocating it for years, and I have thousands of women who can attest to its success.

41. Joyce, in *The Fat-Burning Workout*, you demonstrate how to stand (pose) in a bathing suit and how to wear a bathing suit to one's greatest advantage. I would like to know which bathing suits to avoid altogether, and why.

My heart goes out to the many women I see wearing unflattering suits. "Don't they know that they could look ten pounds lighter in a more flattering style?" I ask myself.

A two-piece *skirt* bathing suit with a loud print, such as polka dots, stripes, or blazing flowers, is probably the worst choice for anyone—fat or thin. The skirt only makes your hips look wider, and the loud print makes you look rounder. If you want to add insult to injury, select such a suit with a skimpy top—one that cannot cover your breasts fully, and let the suit cut across your breasts at the bottom. Then slop a lot of greasy oil all over your stomach and let it all hang out. And, oh, yes—pull the suit down as low as you can; after all, you want to get as tan as possible!

If you have any doubt as to how unflattering such a suit can be, just look at me. I took the photo on the left the same day I took the one on the right, and the other flattering bathing suit photographs in this book. Gee. I'm wondering if I'll win a beauty prize. Let me know if you hear of any contests.

Unflattering bathing suit and pose   *Flattering bathing suit and pose*

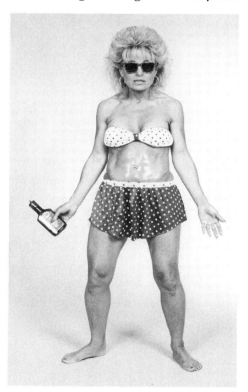
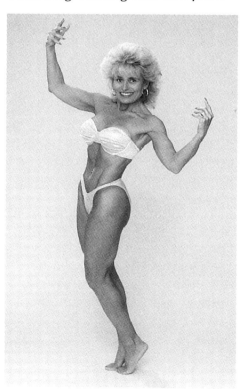

BEFORE I SAY GOOD-BYE

It's not really good-bye. It's really so long, because it will only be as long as it takes for you to write to me before you hear from me again. I'm not going to abandon you. I'm sticking with you all the way. If you have a question or a comment, or if you just need some encouragement, write to me at the address below, and if you include *a stamped, self-addressed envelope*, I will personally answer your letter. Sometimes I write my answer on your letter, other times I type a separate letter to you, depending upon how busy I am. But I always answer—and it's always me and no one else. If you wish to order dumbbells, the bench, the stair stepper, the trampoline, or the mat, use the same address.

Joyce L. Vedral
P.O. Box A 433
Wantagh, NY 11793-0433

Cast-Iron Dumbbells
(as seen in exercise photographs)

Set of three-pound dumbbells, $12.98
Set of five-pound dumbbells, $17.98
Set of eight-pound dumbbells, $24.98
Set of ten-pound dumbbells, $29.98
Set of twelve-pound dumbbells, $34.98
Set of fifteen-pound dumbbells, $39.98
(You pay UPS shipping charges C.O.D.)

Flat-Incline-Decline, Black Upholstered, White Steel Exercise Bench with My Signature.
(as seen in exercise photographs; not sold in stores)
$149.98 plus $19.02 shipping and handling, for a total of $169.00. (Shipped UPS, fully paid.)

BMI Stepper with Multifunction Electronic Monitor
(as seen in photograph on page 194)
$149.98 plus $19.02 shipping and handling, for a total of $169.00. (Shipped UPS, fully paid.)

284

BMI 38″ Low-Impact Aerobic Trampoline
This heavy-gauge steel tube–constructed trampoline is made with heavy-duty springs and durable blue vinyl (as seen on page 194). $49.98 plus $12.02 shipping and handling for a total price of $62.00. (Shipped UPS, fully paid.)

24″-by-68″ Vinyl Exercise Mat with My Signature and Personal Saying: "Feminine muscularity for the women of the nineties."
(as seen in exercise photographs; not sold in stores)
$29.98 plus $8.02 shipping and handling for a total of $38.00. (Shipped UPS, fully paid.)

BIBLIOGRAPHY

NUTRITION, DIET, AND COOKBOOKS

Katahn, Martin, Ph.D., Jamie Pope Cordle, M.S., *The T-Factor Fat Gram Counter.* New York: W. W. Norton & Company, 1989.

Kirshbaum, John (ed.). *The Nutrition Almanac.* New York: McGraw-Hill, 1989.

Natow, Annette B., Ph.D., R.D., and Jo-Ann Heslin, M.A., R.D. *The Fat Attack Plan.* New York: Pocket Books, 1990.

Pritikin: *Pritikin Cookbook* 3d ed. Los Angeles: Pritikin Systems, Inc., 1989.

Reynolds, Bill, and Joyce L. Vedral, Ph.D. *Supercut: Nutrition for the Ultimate Physique.* Chicago: Contemporary Books, 1987.

OTHER FITNESS BOOKS AND VIDEOS AUTHORED AND COAUTHORED BY JOYCE L. VEDRAL

Vedral, Joyce L., Ph.D. *The Fat-Burning Workout.* New York: Warner Books, 1991. (Also available in video: *The Fat-Burning Workout,* Volume I and Volume II, at all video stores.)

Vedral, Joyce L., Ph.D. *Gut Busters.* New York: Warner Books, 1992.

286

Vedral, Joyce L., Ph.D., *Now or Never.* New York: Warner Books, 1986.

Vedral, Joyce L., Ph.D. *The 12-Minute Total-Body Workout.* New York: Warner Books, 1989.

Kneuer, Cameo, and Joyce L. Vedral, Ph.D. *Cameo Fitness.* New York: Warner Books, 1990.

McLish, Rachel, and Joyce L. Vedral, Ph.D. *Perfect Parts.* New York: Warner Books, 1987.

Portuguese, Gladys, and Joyce L. Vedral, Ph.D. *Hard Bodies Express Workout.* New York: Dell Publishing Company, 1988.

Portuguese, Gladys, and Joyce L. Vedral, Ph.D. *Hard Bodies.* New York: Dell Publishing Company, 1986.

Weider, Betty, and Joyce L. Vedral, Ph.D. *Better and Better.* New York: Dell Publishing, Company 1993.

SELF-HELP BOOKS AUTHORED BY JOYCE L. VEDRAL

For Women

Get Rid of Him. New York: Warner Books, 1993.

For Parents

My Teenager Is Driving Me Crazy. New York: Ballantine Books, 1989.

For Teens

Boyfriends: Getting Them, Keeping Them, Living without Them. New York: Ballantine Books, 1990.
I Can't Take It Anymore. New York: Ballantine Books, 1988.
I Dare You. New York: Ballantine Books, 1983.
My Parents Are Driving Me Crazy. New York: Ballantine Books, 1986.
My Teacher Is Driving Me Crazy. New York: Ballantine Books, 1991.
The Opposite Sex Is Driving Me Crazy. New York: Ballantine Books, 1988.
Teens Are Talking: The Question Game for Teens. New York: Ballantine Books, 1993.

The parent book and all of the teen books can be ordered by calling 1-800-733-3000. The other Vedral books can be found in or ordered from your local bookstore.

INDEX